NAIL THE BOARDS !
THE ULTIMATE INTERNAL MEDICINE REVIEW FOR BOARD EXAMS

Bradley D. Mittman, M.D.

D1475851

FIRST EDITION

Frontrunners Board Review, Inc.
56-44 Francis Lewis Blvd.
Bayside, NY 11364

Publisher's Cataloguing-in-Publication
(Provided by Quality Books, Inc.)

Mittman, Bradley D.
   Nail the Boards! : the ultimate internal medicine review for board
exams / Bradley D. Mittman—1st ed.

p. cm.
      Includes bibliographical references and index.
      LCCN: 00-132303
      ISBN: 0-9677025-2-6

1. Internal medicine—Outlines, syllabi, etc.
2. Internal medicine—Examinations, questions, etc.
3. American Board of Internal Medicine—Examinations.
4. Internists—Certification and recertification. I. Title.

      RC58.M58 2000   616'.0076
                                       QBI00-455

PREFACE

This review is aimed at practicing internists and residents of internal medicine who have been searching for a concise, outlined, and one-of-a-kind review of internal medicine for the ABIM certification and recertification exams *as well as* the internal medicine components of other boards exams, including the USMLE, FLEX, and national exams. Designed with the boards in mind, this book is an excellent *companion* to the Frontrunners' Q&A Review for the I.M. Boards, which features *1,234 Q&A* to prepare you for battle. At the same time these resources are outstanding study aids for medical students, residents, internists, and other health care professionals who simply want the *best* no-nonsense review of internal medicine. Originally designed as the syllabus for the Frontrunners Internal Medicine Board Review Course, currently being held in Queens, New York, this book remains today much of the same core material for the board review course, which has seen unparalleled pass rates among its students on the boards. Over the years, we've been blessed with tons of questions and answers from the boards that have been voluntarily submitted by physicians, who have gone on to pass the ABIM exam, in their effort to help those "soldiers left behind"! The course has been widely and enthusiastically received for its highly realistic, "know this" approach to the review of internal medicine. Unfortunately, thousands of physicians, wanting to be board-certified, are simply unable to attend a formal board review course due to time or geographic constraints. For those physicians especially this book will be a welcome review.

All major subsections of the exam have been represented with each section bearing its own chapter. Aren't you tired of reading and rereading (or even falling asleep!) amid long-winded paragraphs from standard textbooks that never make it clear what's important to know for the exam? So were we, and that's how this syllabus came into being. This book is completely outlined making it much more readable since the relationship between concepts is crystal clear—no more guessing! You'll also find tons of *excellent mnemonics* that you'll definitely want to use on your boards along with contributive formatting through the use of bolds, underlining, italics, boxed-in points, and starred items ✪ to help call attention to *particularly* important material, although we would like to think that everything in here is important. Moreover, the convenient *Index section* will make those quick look-ups a breeze.

Having said all this, we also realize that there are individuals who have, over the years, grown weary of tedious self-study and who want to take advantage of our more formal sit-down, or "feed-me" style of board review, with much the same core material, but featuring tons of key slides, cases, Xrays, EKGs, and more. For this reason we continue to hold our formal board review courses, which include: 1) the *Weekend Marathon* board review courses offered throughout the year, typically a few weeks before the exam—ideal for most physicians who can only spare a weekend; that weekend, however, covers 16 hours of highly intensive review and is not for the faint of heart; and 2) our more detailed 4-month board review course for more local physicians. For details/registration on any of our internal medicine board review courses or to order the *Frontrunners Q&A Review for the I.M. Boards: 1,234 Q&A to Prepare You*, call us at 888-440-2246.

Most would agree that being a great physician and passing the exam are not at all synonymous. Unfortunately, HMOs *would not* agree. In fact, HMOs are requiring that their PCPs be board-certified, or, at the very least, board-eligible to come on-board and *stay* on-board. In fact, the terms "board-certified" and "board-eligible" are increasingly becoming an integral part of HMO contracts and renewal criteria. Being board-certified, therefore, is no longer a luxury. To some physicians, passing the exam means more than just placating the HMOs or even maintaining one's practice. It's about personal challenge; it's about being able to call oneself a "board-certified internist"; but even more simply, it's about *winning*! We want *you* to win.

We're confident that you'll find this an outstanding resource for your upcoming board exam as well as your day-to-day practice of internal medicine. But however you plan to use this book, our greatest hope is that we help you achieve your goals and make your life a whole lot easier!

With best wishes for you,

Bradley D. Mittman, MD

Bradley D. Mittman, MD
FRONTRUNNERS BOARD REVIEW, INC.

• NOTICE •

This book is designed as primarily as a study aid for the American Board of Internal Medicine certification and recertification exams. It was originally designed and remains the core of the syllabus for the Frontrunners Board Review, Inc. internal medicine board review course. The book is not intended to serve as a complete or standard textbook of internal medicine nor any subspecialties, but rather as a resource to assist the physician in his or her review specifically for the exam. It is in no way intended to be used as the sole reference for one's study or practice of internal medicine nor any subspecialties. Neither the author nor the publisher can be held accountable for any student's or students' individual board scores, as it is expected that all students will invest significant time in personal review of this and other materials such as general textbooks of medicine.

Medicine is an ever-changing science. As new research and clinical experience broaden our knowledge, changes in the treatment and drug therapy are required The author and publisher of this work have checked with sources believed to be reliable in their efforts to provide information that is complete and generally in accord with the standards accepted at the time of publication. However, in view of the possibility of human error or changes in medical sciences, neither the author nor the publisher nor any other party who has been involved in the preparation or publication of this work warrants that the information contained herein is in every respect accurate or complete, and they are not responsible for any errors or omissions or for the results obtained from use of such information. Readers are encouraged to confirm the information contained herein with other sources. This is particularly true insofar as drug selection and dosage are concerned. The reader is urged to check the package insert for each drug for any change in indications or contraindications, dosage, warnings, precautions, or drug-drug interactions.

Dedication

To Andre without whom this work
would never have come to be.
"You're my star, and when I'm far,
you're not alone, 'cause your heart's
my home."--Lenny Kravitz

TABLE OF CONTENTS:

1. <u>HEMATOLOGY</u>

Commonly Asked Material:

1. Know the differential diagnosis for <u>**Isolated Thrombocytosis (plt>400)**</u>

   a) Essential Thrombocythemia
   b) Transitory Thrombocytosis
      i. Exercise
      ii. Stress
      iii. Epinephrine
   c) *Reactive thrombocytosis*
      i. Malignancy
      ii. Post-op (splenectomy; post-op stress)
      iii. Inflammatory disorders
      iv. Acute hemorrhage
      v. Fe def. anemia
      vi. P. Vera
      vii. Hemolytic anemia
      viii. Idiopathic myelofibrosis

2. Know that <u>**Waldenstrom's Macroglobulinemia**</u> is IgM, and know the presentation.

   - A lymphoproliferative disorder of excess IgM production, yielding presentations of either splenomegaly and anemia, or hyperviscosity-related symptoms, such as headache, chest pain, SOB, fatigue, and lethargy.

3. Can <u>**Pernicious Anemia**</u> lead to malignancy?

   - Yes, the disease develops into malignancy in **10%** of cases.

4. Recognize a classic case of <u>**TTP**</u> (Thrombotic Thrombocytopenic Purpura) and know the initial management:

   ✪ Remember: "<u>F.A.T. R.N.</u>" to recall the classic pentad of presenting signs and symptoms:

   > **F**ever
   > **A**nemia (microangiopathic hemolytic anemia); hemolysis→ *schistocytes*
   > **T**hrombocytopenia
   > **R**enal findings
   > **N**eurologic findings

   - Etiology: 90% are idiopathic; most of the rest are seen with pregnancy and OCPs
   - Coombs *negative*
   - Treatment of choice is plasmapheresis, using FFP plasma exchange

5. Be able to recognize a Schistocyte/**Schistocytes** on a peripheral blood smear and know the entire DDx

> ✪ **AGN, ARF, DIC, HTN, Pulm HTN, HUS, PAN, SLE, TTP, HELLP syndrome, and preeclampsia**→all of these can give microangiopathic hemolytic anemia (**Coombs negative**)→which in turn gives *schistocytes*

6. Know **Autoimmune Hemolysis**

- You order a **Coombs test** (also known as D.A.T. or Direct Antiglobulin Test) when you suspect AHA. Accordingly, a positive Coombs test means the hemolytic anemia is *immune*. The term "direct", as in "His Direct Coombs test was positive" implies detection of antibodies *directly* on the RBC membrane. The following chart is useful in helping you distinguish warm (70%) vs. cold (15%) antibodies. The remainder of the antibodies are drug-induced (so-called "Coombs-negative AHA").

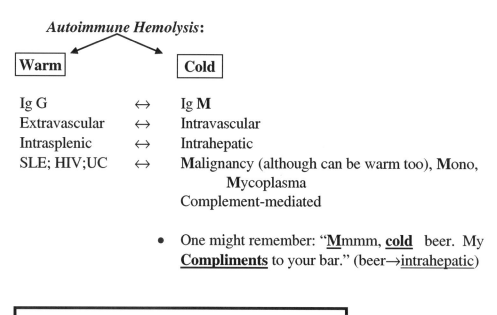

Autoimmune Hemolysis:

Warm		Cold
Ig G	↔	Ig **M**
Extravascular	↔	Intravascular
Intrasplenic	↔	Intrahepatic
SLE; HIV;UC	↔	Malignancy (although can be warm too), **M**ono, **M**ycoplasma
		Complement-mediated

- One might remember: "**M**mmm, **cold** beer. My **Compliments** to your bar." (beer→intrahepatic)

> - See Figure 1 (Appendix): Hemolytic Anemia--Algorithm

7. **Know to order a Peripheral Blood Smear in someone who presents with thrombocytopenia (<150) for the first time**.

- The peripheral blood smear is valuable for two main reasons here: 1) in order to R/O plt clumping (which can give you falsely lower platelet counts; and 2) if platelets are truly low on the PBS, a bone marrow biopsy will be needed to check for megakaryocytes (platelet precursors), which, if elevated, imply peripheral platelet loss/consumption, and, if low, imply underproduction of platelets by the bone marrow.

> - See Figure 2 (Appendix): Thrombocytopenia--Algorithm

8. Be able to recognize **Fe-Deficiency Anemia** on a peripheral blood smear. Remember the central pallor combined with an erythrocyte size comparable to the size of a surrounding normal lymphocyte nucleus.

9. **CML:**

   a) **Know WHEN TO USE hydroxyurea (Hydrea) and alpha interferon**
      i. Blast crisis
      ii. Leukocytosis
      iii. All patients considered candidates for bone marrow transplant since they cannot receive Busulfan 2° to risk of:
         a)) **Interstitial pneumonitis**
         b)) **Veno-occlusive disease** (VOD)
      iv. Re: hydroxyurea and alpha interferon as well as anegrelide can also be used to treat essential thrombocytosis.

   b) **Be able to recognize a CML CBC differential:**
      i. Leukocytosis >100,000 common; <10% blasts in chronic phase
      ii. Granulocytes seen in all stages of maturation with basophilia and eosinophilia
      iii. Platelets often > 400,000

   c) **Know the CML translocation:**
      i. The Philadelphia chromosome (**t 9,22**) is the hallmark of the disease
      ii. The Philadelphia chromosome carries a *good* prognosis, as opposed to AML (poor prognosis)
      iii. ✪ This *translocation* results in the formation of a **chimeric bcr-abl gene** resulting in:
         a)) Maturation block (granulocytes) as noted above on the peripheral blood smear
         b)) Blast crisis

   d) **Know when the CML patient who would benefit from a bone marrow transplant (BMT)**
      • Allogeneic BMT should be performed during the chronic phase, within the first 6-12 months in patients < 55 y.o. who have an HLA-identical match or an identical twin.

10. Understand the indication for *Autologous* BMT

    • It is used preferred when the patient's bone marrow is normal and we want to remove the marrow and spare it from the highly bone marrow-toxic chemotherapeutic regimens of such cancers as germ cell tumors and breast cancer, after which regimens the patient's original normal marrow may be returned to the patient without having suffered the toxicity.

11. **Treatment of Blood Product** → **In order to prevent**

    • Washed/frozen RBCs — Febrile/allergic reactions
    • Irradiation — GVHD (Graft vs. Host Disease)
    • 3rd generation filter (leukocyte depleted) — CMV

12. Patients with **bleeding diathesis**:

    a) If the PTT does not "correct" on a "**1 to 1 dilution test**" ✪ (aka "mixing study", where patient serum is mixed with control serum that should have all the appropriate clotting factors), then there is an inhibitor present (e.g. Factor VIII inhibitor, lupus anticoagulant, anticardiolipin antibody, etc).

    b) Know the important differences between **von Willebrand Dz** and **Hemophilia**

	<u>Hemophilia A</u> vs.	<u>vWD</u>
Bleeding time	*Normal*	*Prolonged*
Inheritance	Sex-linked	Autosomal
Factor 8 rag	Normal	↓
Ristocetin	Normal	↓

> ✪ <u>**Coagulation**</u> **disorders**: These are characterized by joint, soft tissue and organ bleeding.
> ✪ **Defects in** <u>**platelet function**</u>: These are characterized by purpura (petechiae and ecchymoses) of the skin and hemorrhage from mucous membranes.

    c) Know the <u>**indications for FFP**</u> (fresh frozen plasma)

        i. FFP has all blood factors except 5 & 8, so can use for most everything, except must use cryoprecipitate for Hemophilia A

        ii. **Useful in multiple coagulation disorders:**

            ◆ Anticoagulation overdose
            ◆ Liver disease
            ◆ Massive transfusion
            ◆ DIC
            ◆ Plasmaphereses
            ◆ Vit K deficiency

        ✪ <u>**KEY ANTIPHOSPHOLIPID SYNDROMES**</u> (*factor inhibitors* which ↑ **PTT**)

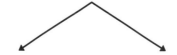

Lupus Anticoagulant
(This is a <u>*pro*</u>coagulant!)
                Anticardiolipin Antibody

Common DDx of Lupus Anticoagulant
1. SLE
2. ITP
3. RA
4. AIDS
5. *Drugs*: Dilantin, Hydralazine
   Quinidine, Procainamide

See Figure 3 (Appendix):　　　　**Intrinsic & Extrinsic Clotting Cascade**

	↑ **PTT**	Normal PTT
↑**PT**	↓ 2,5,10	↓ 7 ↓vit K (malnutrition)
Normal PT	↓12 (no bleeding) ↓11 (mild bleeding) ↓8,9 (severe bleed)	↓13

13. Recognize a case of **Delayed Transfusion Reaction:** i.e. 3-5 days after receiving a transfusion of packed red blood cells, the patient returns to the hospital with **scleral icterus, malaise, fatigue, elevated LDH**, etc.
    a. Incidence: F>M
    b. Cause: Antibody in the *recipient vs. foreign-donor serum proteins*. The recipient's plasma already contains antibody before the transfusion because of previous transfusion, or previous pregnancy.
    c. *Coombs test is +*
    d. 1/3rd of these reactions are asymptomatic. The rest may show *Fever/Chills/Jaundice/Anemia*
    e. **Treatment**…
        i. IV fluids
        ii. Give antihistamines
        iii. Monitor Hb and urine output

14. Know that **recurrent abortions may be seen in**:
    a. *Anticardiolipin syndrome*
    b. *Lupus anticoagulant*
    c. *Fibrinogen disorders*
    d. *Factor 13 deficiency*

15. Be able to recognize **atypical lymphocytes**, *associated with mononucleosis*, on a peripheral blood smear.

16. Recognize a classic case of **H.A.T.T. (Heparin Associated Thrombocytopenia with Thrombosis)**

    a) Incidence varies anywhere from 1-30%

    b) Heparin may enhance platelet aggregation, causing:
- Decrease platelet count
- Thrombosis (venous > arterial)

    c) The mechanism is immunologic, with heparin-specific Ig G and antibodies vs. the platelet-heparin complex

    d) **Develops 3-15 days after initiating the heparin, with a median time of 10 days** after initiation.

    e) The treatment is to stop the heparin ASAP (similar to above with delayed transfusion reactions)

    f) Because of HATT, a CBC should be checked QD in patients on heparin, with special attention to the platelets.

HEMATOLOGY NOTES

HYPOCHROMIC MICROCYTIC ANEMIAS:

Disease	MCV	RBCs	RDW	TIBC	Fe	Ferritin
Fe deficiency anemia	↓	↓	>16	↑ (<15)	↓	↓
Anemia of chronic dz	↓ or nl	↓	↑	(>15) or nl	↓	↑ or nl
Thalassemia minor	↓	↑	<16	nl	nl/↑	↑ or nl

THALASSEMIA

- ◆ Defective globin chain synthesis, therefore defective Hgb
- ◆ Can affect the alpha or the beta chains, and can be minor (heterozygous) or major (homozygous)
- ◆ *Beta thalassemia* (2 genes) can be either heterozygous ("trait"), showing microcytosis with mild or no anemia, or homozygous, showing severe anemia
- ◆ *Alpha thalassemia* involves 4 genes. If only one is affected, the disease is usually silent. If 2 genes are affected, see microcytosis. A 3 gene defect yields Hgb H disease. Defects in all 4 genes yields hydrops fetalis.
- ✪ B. thalassemia: look for ↑ **Hgb A2** on Hgb electropheresis (normal 2.5%; 5% in B Thal major and minor)
- ◆ B. thal. **major**
  - ✪ Look for ↑ **Fetal Hgb** (normal < 1%; 50% in Thal major; 2-3% in Thal minor)
  - • B. thalassemia major rarely survives to adulthood without BMT
- ◆ Electropheresis is normal in alpha thalassemia
- ◆ *B. thalassemia minor is the predominant thalassemia seen in adults*
  - • presents asymptomatically with a microcytic-hypochromic anemia

ERYTHROPOETIN LEVELS

- • Re: there is an inverse relationship between the epo level and the Hgb (or Hct). Regulation is linked to an oxygen sensor.

↓ Epo level	↑ Epo level
P. Vera	Pure RBC aplasia
R.A.	Fe deficiency
HIV	Tumors (esp renal)
	High altitude

✪ IMPORTANT CELL TYPES ON PERIPHERAL BLOOD SMEAR:

- **Ringed sideroblasts**→alcohol is the #1 cause of aquired sideroblastic anemia

- **Spherocytes**→autoimmune hemolytic anemia

- **Atypical (reactive) lymphocyte**→infectious mono

- **Basophilic stippling**→ *thalassemia*, arsenic, lead poisoning

- **Target cells**→ *thalassemia*, jaundice/hepatitis, post-splenectomy

- **Stomatocytes**→acute alcoholism; hereditary hemolytic anemia

- **Acanthocytes** (Spur cells)→liver disease

- **Burr cells**→Uremia, DIC

- **Heinz bodies**→G6PD deficiency (*Coombs-positive* hemolysis); **Italian & African-American** men
  - Key culprits (drugs)→antimalarials; sulfonamides; dapsone; nitrofurantoin; nitrites

- **Helmet cells=Schistocytes** (from any cause of microangiopathic hemolytic anemia—see DDx above in question section)→*Coombs test is negative*

- **Auer rods**→PML (Promyelocytic leukemia=AML M3 subtype); if you have to have AML, hope to see Auer rods, since M3 carries the best prognosis 2° to treatment options with ATRA (all-transretinoic acid)

- **Hairy cells**→Hairy cell leukemia (curable with 2CDA); these cells are said to have a "fried egg" appearance.

PAROXYSMAL NOCTURNAL HEMOGLOBINURIA

1. PNH is a chronic disease caused by an unknown idiopathic defect in the RBC

2. 50% of deaths due to PNH are associated with ***venous thromboembolism***, including Hepatic V Thrombosis (**Budd-Chiari Syndrome** is the major cause of death)

3. *Hemolysis is intravascular, yielding Hgbemia and Hgburia*

4. Leukemia (**AML**) develops in 5-10%

5. *Aplastic anemia* is an important complication to remember for the exam

6. Dx: *Ham test and sucrose hemolysis test*

HEREDITARY SPHEROCYTOSIS

1. Occurs 2° to a defect in the RBC membrane cytoskeleton component called spectrin
2. Splenomegaly
3. Coombs negative
4. Tx→splenectomy

VITAMIN B12 DEFICIENCY

1. KEY FEATURES:
    a) *Hypersegmented neutrophils*; important sign as often appear before the:

       (1) **Macrocytosis**; or
       (2) **Anemia (megaloblastic),** which can also result from folate deficiency

    b) ↑ *Serum MMA* (methylmalonic acid) level; ↑ serum gastrin levels.

    c) *Schilling test* important for finding the cause

    d) *Pernicious anemia*

       (1) The #1 cause of Vitamin B12 deficiency
       (2) Check **anti-intrinsic factor (IF) antibodies** in the serum for diagnosis
       (3) Check TFTs as thyroid disorders, also ↑ incidence of hyper or Hypothyroidism (other autoimmine disorders)
       (4) ↑ risk of gastric malignancy, so consider direct visualization and biopsy with endoscopy

    e) *Neurologic findings*

       (1) Ataxic gait 2° to degeneration of the posterior columns
       (2) Dementia
       (3) Seizures

2. TYPICAL ORDER of events in B12 deficiency…

    a) Serum homocysteine and MMA ↑
    b) Serum B12 ↓
    c) MCV ↑ but still normal; hypersegmented neutrophils seen
    d) MCV ↑ beyond normal
    e) Anemia develops
    f) Symptoms seen

✪ Note that while this is the *usual* sequence of events, patients symptomatic with B12 deficiency ***need not have*** abnormal MCV or Hct !

FOLATE DEFICIENCY

1. Usually secondary to poor PO intake (some elderly; dementia); alcoholics; malnutrition
2. *Megaloblastic* anemia as per vit B12 deficiency
3. As opposed to vit B12, however, ***no neurologic complications.***

ALCOHOLISM

1. #1 cause of acquired sideroblastic anemia
2. Can see ↑ MCV (may be 2° to folate defiency)
3. Often see ↑ PT 2° to ↓ production of clotting factors 2° to liver disease

HEMOLYTIC UREMIC SYNDROME (HUS)

1. ✪ Similar to TTP, except w/o the Fever or Neurologic involvement (**FAT R**N without the F or N)

2. Management in adults, however, is the same as for TTP

3. *Hemorrhagic colitis* 2° to **Ecoli 0157H7** (tainted beef)

SICKLE CELL ANEMIA

1. 8% of blacks carry the Sickle cell **trait;**

2. Patients with sickle cell **trait** often have painless **hematuria** and may be associated with pyelonephritis in pregnancy; there is **no anemia, no ↑ risk of infections, no ↑ mortality;** those with "trait" also have difficulty concentrating their urine (hypo/isosthenuria). They have no pain crises.

3. Long-term exchange transfusion in SS anemia useful in patients with **cerebrovascular complications;**

4. **Treatment**→Prevention; Hydration; Analgesia; Exchange Transfusions as appropriate to decrease the Hgb S to <30%) ; ***Hydrea*** used to ↓ risk of complications;

5. **Pathophysiology**→Acute crises are due to recurrent obstruction of the microcirculation by intravascular sickling, caused by diminished oxygen delivery→more sickling→worse oxygen delivery→etc.

6. **Atypical symptoms** may suggest→pneumonia; pulmonary infarction; acute pyelonephritis; or cholecystitis. Remember, infections are the #1 cause of death in SS disease;

7. **5 *Main* Crises ✪ :**

   a) **Vaso-occlusive("painful" or "infarctive" crisis)**
      i) Most frequent type of crisis
      ii) 2° to microvascular obstruction from sickled cells which starts the cycle of tissue hypoxia that in turn causes more sickling.
      iii) Seen in long bones, chest, and abdomen
      iv) Causes autosplenectomy

   b) **Aplastic Crisis**
      i) Bone marrow suppression 2° to infections (usually viral)
      ii) Because of the short RBC lifespan, even brief periods of suppression may have a significant effect on Hgb level
      iii) Usually follows a febrile illness and lasts 5-10 days

   c) **Megaloblastic Crisis**
      i) Usually due to folate deficiency, esp in late pregancy
      ii) Associated with ↑MCV and ↓Hgb

   d) **Sequestration Crisis**
      i) Pooling of RBCs in the spleen, seen primarily in young children

   e) **Hemolytic Crisis**
      i) Usually 2° to infection or drugs→ ↑retic count, ↑unconjugated bili, and jaundice
      ii) Especially in patients with G6PD deficiency, hereditary spherocytosis, and mycoplasma pneumonia

8. <u>Avascular necrosis</u> a common complication; remember to order the MRI if you suspect it!

9. **Renal complications→papillary necrosis; <u>hyposthenuria</u>** (inability to concentrate the urine; nocturia; enuresis); focal segmental glomerulonephropathy;

10. **Priapism** also common;

11. ✪ **Pulmonary** Crisis: <u>**Acute Chest Syndrome**</u> causes 20% of SS deaths: look for Fever, Chest pain, Tachypnea, ↑WBC count, and pulmonary infarcts; in adults sickling here is usually unaccompanied by infection.

CLL (Chronic Lymphocytic Leukemia)

1. **#1** malignancy in the U.S. and #1 form of leukemia ≥60 yo; 90% of pts are > 50 yo; CLL is characterized by malignant B lymphocytes.

2. **Fever** should always be presumed 2° to infection and not the leukemia (except for ***Richter's transformation to Large Cell Lymphoma, which carries a poor prognosis***)

3. ↓ **Gamma globulins** (re: CLL is a disease of B cells) predispose to infection. Of those with infection, half have low gamma globulins

4. Other **complications**→Autoimmune hemolytic anemia; thrombocytopenia; ↑incidence of solid tumors of the lung and skin; AML

5. A poor prognosticator is **lymphocyte doubling time** in < 1 year

6. ✪ Staging: <u>**Rai classification**</u>:

    Stage 0:   Lymphocytosis only
    Stage 1:   "   + Lymphadenopathy
    Stage 2:   "   +   "   +   Splenomegaly

    Stage 3:   "   **+ Anemia**
    Stage 4:   "   **+ Thrombocytopenia**

---

7. ✪ Remember it's important to know the Rai stage since <u>treatment does not prolong survival</u> in <u>stages I or II</u>, and is generally **reserved for Stage 3 and 4 only**! *Management* of Rai 3 (+ anemia) and Rai 4 (+ thrombocytopenia) includes <u>chlorambucil ± prednisone</u>. For patients who relapse, <u>fludarabine</u> is often used.

---

8. **Gamma globulin therapy** may be given prophylatically even if the patient has never had infection, as long as his Ig G is <0.3 g/dl.

9. The **median survival time** for CLL is 5 years from the onset of treatment.

HAIRY CELL LEUKEMIA

1. Represents < 2% of all leukemia; cytopenias/splenomegaly predominate; essentially a B cell dz.

2. **<u>Hairy cells ("fried egg" appearance)</u>** with cytoplasmic projections seen on blood smears

3. **<u>TRAP +</u>** (stain positively to tartrate-resistant acid phosphatase)

4. **<u>Dry TAP</u>** on bone marrow aspiration (consistent with the pancytopenia often seen)

5. ✪ Neutropenia→infections (these infections are different as they tend to be **<u>atypical mycobacterial and other ususual infections, like toxoplasmosis, legionella, and nocardia</u>**)→these infections are the primary cause of mortality in HCL.

6. ✪ **<u>2CDA is the treatment</u>** of choice, producing complete remission in 85%-88% of patients after a single continuous 7day IV infusion.

HODGKIN'S DISEASE

1. Central to the diagnosis is the presence of the **Reed-Sternberg cell**, a large cell with a bilobed or multilobulated nucleus with prominent inclusion-like nucleoli, giving the appearance of "owl's eyes."
2. 1/5 to ½ have EBV in their genome
3. Remember, the *staging is based on SITES ON INVOLVEMENT*, not on the histology
4. **XRT** is the Rx of choice for Stages 1-3A1; **Chemo** is for Stage 3A2, Stage 3B, and Stage 4. ✪
5. **Long term complications of chemotherapy** include AML, Solid Tumors, and Diffuse Aggressive Lymphomas. ✪

NHL (Non-Hodgkin's Lymphoma)

1. Remember, the *staging is based on HISTOLOGY*
2. NHL patients fall into one of 3 categories

    i)   **Low Grade**—*very responsive to initial tx; yet, not curable*
          a)   Multiple Myeloma
          b)   Waldenstrom's Macroglobulinema (re:Anemia; Splenomegaly; IgM spike; hyperviscosity sx's)
          c)   CLL
    ii)   **Intermediate--curable**
          •   DLCL (Diffuse Large Cell Lymphoma)
    iii) **High Grade**
          a)   Lymphoblastic
          b)   Immunoblastic
          c)   Burkitt's (ALL3; aka Small non-cleaved)

3. The key **prognosticators** ✪ in NHL are:
          a)   LDH
          b)   Age (>60)
          c)   Stage (3,4)
          d)   Performance status
          e)   Bulk of disease

---

4   Remember, as you go from Less mature→→→→More mature, you also go from high grade lymphomas→→→low grade lymphomas.

---

5. High Grades—additional points:
          a)   Often see Neurologic involvement
          b)   Allogeneic BMT following remission
          c)   ↑↑LDH and U.A. and low phos
          d)   30-40% survival for all comers
          e)   "Leukemic" when bone marrow involved

vi).   <u>ABVD</u>   =   <u>CHOP</u>
      Hodgkin's   Non-Hodgkin's

MULTIPLE MYELOMA ✪

1. **≥10% plasma cells found in the bone marrow**   { **< 10% in MGUS** (Monoclonal Gammopathy of Undetermined Significance) }

2. **M protein→ < 3 g/dl in MGUS; > 3 in MM**

3. Clinical features→<u>bone pain (#1 symptom)</u>; renal insufficiency; <u>hypercalcemia</u>; weakness/fatigue; **spinal cord compression; pneumococcal infection**.

4. Normochromic normocytic anemia

5. Xrays→*<u>"punched out" lytic lesions</u>*; osteoporosis; pathologic **fractures**

6. Because it is not curable, tx should be delayed until evidence of progression seen.

AML (Acute Myelogenous Leukemia=Acute Nonlymphocytic Leukemia, ANLL)

1. Remember, the **Philadelphia** chromosome (t 9,22), carries a *worse* **prognosis** here (**as opposed to CML**)

2. Age <40 yo and achieving complete remission after first cycle of Idarubicin (or Daunarubicin) + AraC (Cytarabine) carry good prognosis.

3. For patients who present with with acute leukemia who present with **WBC>100,000** the initial complication of greatest concern is cerebral hemorrhage.

     <u>EMERGENCY TREATMENT INCLUDES:</u>
         a)   **Hydration**
         b)   **Hydrea**
         c)   **Alkalinization of the urine**
         d)   **Allopurinol**
         e)   **Radiation**
         f)   **Leukopheresis**

4. Median age of patients with AML is 65 yo

5. Platelet transfusions are required throughout the course of treatment.

6. Recommendations:
   - *If patient <55yo →consider BMT in 1st remission if poor prognostic; BMT in early relapse or 2nd remission if no poor prognostics.*

AML Response to Chemo Alone:

AML
↓
Idarubicin (or Daunarubicin) + Ara C
↓
55-85% achieve remission (90% in M3)
↓
Most relapse within 1 year
↓
2nd remission can be achieved in 30-50%
↓
Ultimately only a 20% survival rate

ALL (Acute Lymphoblastic Leukemia)

1. More common in **children** (who have complete remission rates of >90%)

2. 1/3 of patients present with **bleeding**

3. Bone pain/LN/HM/SM are more common in ALL (3/4 patients) than AML (1/2 of patients)

4. **CALLa antigen** is a **good** prognosticator

THE MYELOPROLIFERATIVE DISORDERS :

The four disorders—ALL can lead to AML!   *LAP Score*

1. **CML--**   ↑**WBCs**   ↓

2. **Myelofibrosis--**   ↑**Fibrosis**   ↑

3. **P. Vera --**   ↑**RBCs**   ↑

4. **1° Thrombocythemia--**   ↑**Platelets**   ↑

- *Other disorders with ↓ LAP scores* include: PNH, aplastic anemia, and Wilson's

Let's examine each of the main myeloproliferative disorders one by one…

1. CML:

- **Philadelphia chromosome** (t 9,22) is the hallmark
  - *translocation causes a bcr-abl chimeric gene→results in premature termination of granulocyte maturation and also results in blast crisis.*

- **The only *low* LAP score among the four Myeloproliferative disorders** shown

- An acquired defect of clonal origin

- **CBC→WBC>100,000; granulocytes found in all stages of maturation**; platelets typically>400,000

- Good prognosis→ small spleen size and 0%-10% circulating blasts

- Poor prognosis: age>45 and platelet<70,000

- **Chronic phase**
  - *≤10% blasts in blood and bone marrow*
  - *2-3 years in duration*

- Bone marrow exam reveals
  - hyperplasia
  - 10-40% have myelofibrosis

- ↑ Vit B12, as with P. Vera

- **Treatment**:

  - **Allo BMT is the treatment of choice** and is the only curative regimen, *not* conventional chemo.

    - **Should be performed in the chronic phase , within the 1st 6-12 months in patients <55 yo who have an HLA-identical match or an identical twin.**

    - Survival is 63% at 3 years

  - However, **3 agents commonly used in the initial tx of CML** are:

    1. Hydroxyurea—tx of choice for high blast counts and leukostasis; safe in thrombocytopenia; continued maintenance tx is important.

    2. Busulfan

    3. Alpha interferon—suppresses the Philadelphia chromosome

- Hydroxyurea and alpha interferon are used when the patient will be going for BMT 2° to the greater **TOXICITY OF BUSULFAN**, which can cause:

  1. Interstitial pneumonitis
  2. VOD (veno-occlusive disease)

- Remember the ***COMPLICATIONS of BMT*** in general:

  1. *Early*:

     (1) **GVHD**
         - (a) Skin→rash
         - (b) GI →diarrhea; liver pathology
         - (c) CMV infection
     (2) **V.O.D. (Veno-occlusive disease)**
         - (a) Hepatomegaly
         - (b) Ascites
         - (c) Jaundice

  2. *Late:*
     - (1) HSV, VZV
     - (2) PCP
     - (3) Chronic GVHD

- **MGMT OF "BLAST CRISIS"**→ allopurinol, fluids, hydroxyurea, cranial radiation, and leukocyte apheresis.

✪ **CHRONIC phase→ACCELERATED phase ("BLAST CRISIS") when ≥ 20% BLASTS**

| 2. MYELOFIBROSIS: |

a. *Splenomegaly **always** present*

b. **Hypocellular marrow** 2° replacement of marrow by fibrosis

c. **"Teardrop" cells**

d. Leukoerythroblastic peripheral blood smear in 96%

> ## 3. POLYCYTHEMIA VERA ---Everything is ↑ *except* the Epo level !!

- Remember the first step in approaching a high Hct is to obtain a **RBC mass** (↑)

- **Postbathing pruritis**

- ↑ Spleen size seen in 75%→can lead to hemolysis→ ↑LDH

- **↑ LAP** score is used to differentiate it from other forms of erythrocytosis (stress, anoxic, tumor)

- **↓ Epo** level (remember the inverse correlation with Hgb/Hct).

- **Diagnostic criteria**: ↑RBC mass + arterial Oxygen sat>92% + either (splenomegaly or at leas 2 of the following):

    1. WBC >12,000
    2. Platelets > 400,000 --may treat with Anegralide, hydrea, or alpha interferon, or even P32 (phos)
    3. ↑LAP
    4. ↑B12 (re: seen in CML too)

- Consider P Vera if see splenomegaly + absent Fe stores + microcytosis

- Treatment is **phlebotomy** q 2-4 months if asymptomatic. Keep Hct at 42-45

VON WILLEBRAND'S DISEASE

1. #1 inherited bleeding disorder

2. **Prolonged bleeding time (2° to problem with platelet aggregation, not factor deficiency!); therefore, normal PT/PTT.**

3. vWF (**vW Factor) is decreased** , either in number or function (function is checked by the ristocetin factor assay)

    - **vWF is important in platelet aggregation (thus the prolonged bleeding time)** and functions as carrier protein for factor VIII

4. **dDAVP (desmopressin) is the treatment of choice for minor bleeding; factor 8 concentrate or cryoprecipitate (carries 5,8, and fibrinogen) for more serious bleeds.**

DIC (Disseminated Intravascular Coagulopathy)

1. A "*consumptive coagulopathy*" characterized by microvascular clotting secondary to thrombin deposition.
2. Carries a 50-80% mortality
3. **Platelet aggregation results in *thrombocytopenia*, ↓ fibrinogen, and ↑ D-dimers**

4. ↑*PT, PTT*, and thrombin time

5. ↓ Platelet counts and fibrinogen

6. Classic complication of **PML (*AML type M3*, promyelocytic)** ✪

7. *Schistocytes* seen secondary to the microvascular obstruction

8. Thrombosis > bleeding

9. **Sepsis is the #1 cause**

10. Malignancy is the #2 cause

11. **As opposed to liver disease, DIC produces a much greater thrombocytopenia and Factors 7 and 10 are normal in DIC.**

12. Heparin only indicated with evidence of fibrin deposition and thrombosis.

FACTOR XIII DEFICIENCY ✪

1. **Think of this disease when the patient has <u>delayed post-op bleeding</u> (e.g. after dental work when patient returns home and gums bleed later that night).**

2. **All routing <u>clotting tests are normal</u>; however, → *Urease clot solubility* test is positive.**

3. **<u>FFP</u> is the treatment.**

FACTOR V LEIDEN DEFICIENCY ✪

- **Hereditary activated protein C (<u>aPC</u>) resistance**

- *Accounts for <u>30-50% of patients with "idiopathic" venous thrombosis</u> and 20-30% of cases of DVT in patients <45yo*;   present in 2-5% of the general population!

- **Don't forget (!) to look for this disease in women who develop <u>DVT while on OCPs or while pregnant</u>, i.e. in addition to the usual studies of Protein C & S, etc.**

HYPERCOAGUABLE STATES

FACTOR V LEIDEN DEFICIENCY (APC RESISTANCE)—see above

PROTEIN S DEFICIENCY
- More common than protein C deficiency or AT III deficiency.
- A vitamin K-dependent factor that is **required for activated *protein C* anticoagulant activity**. Remember, **activated protein C functions as an anticoagulant by destroying factors 5 and 8** (with the help of protein S)

PROTEIN C DEFICIENCY—Remember, because of its role in destroying factors 5 and 8, a deficiency in Protein C (or S for that matter) will result in a hypercoaguable state. In patients with protein C deficiency, a potential therapeutic complication is the development *of **warfarin-induced skin necrosis***. This cx results from the short half-life of Protein C which warfarin accelerates, causing rapid depletion and a paradoxical worsening of the hypercoaguable state. For this reason, protein C deficient patients should receive ***heparin first***. Note also that because proteins C and S *are **vitamin-K dependent***, a proper diagnosis of protein C or S def cannot be made if the patient is vit-K deficient.

ANTITHROMBIN III DEFICIENCY
- Seen primarily in **nephrotic syndrome** secondary to loss of the protein thru the urine;
- **Renal vein thrombosis** and other DVTs

LUPUS ANTICOAGULANT
- An antiphospholipid antibody (like anticardiolipin antibodies)
- a PTT inhibitor, so the PTT **does not correct on a 1:1 dilution** test
- **False + VDRL**
- Despite the name, lupus "anticoagulant" is **actually a "pro-coagulant"**

DYSFIBRINOGENEMIAS—check thrombin and reptilase times to screen for these

- **When the PT/PTT does correct on a 1:1 dilution test, measuring 3 factors (5,8,9) can distinguish between the 3 most common causes of acquired factor deficiencies: liver disease, DIC, and vitamin K deficiency.**

	Liver Disease	**DIC**	**Vit K ↓**
Factor V	↓	↓	normal
Factor VIII	normal	↓	normal
Factor IX	↓	↓	↓

- *Remember the **vit K-dependent** factors* are…**2,7,9,10, and proteins C&S**

✪ CRYOPRECIPITATE VS. FRESH FROZEN PLASMA:

Cryoprecipitate →	**Contains: 5, 8, 13, vWF, and fibrinogen**
FFP →	**Contains: all except 5, 8**

WARFARIN

1. Afib, routine DVT, CVA→shoot for **INR 2.0-3.0**

2. **Recurrent DVT or mechanical (prosthetic) heart valve→ shoot for INR 3.0-4.5**

3. Contraindicated in pregnancy because of the risk of teratogenesis (nasal hyoplasia; CNS abnormalities)

4. Re: Metronidazole and Sulfonamides: ↑ warfarin level
   Barbiturates, Carbamazapine, and Rifampin: ↓ warfarin level

Warfarin Interactions with Commonly Used Meds: *COUMADIN PACT*:

    C ardiac drugs: amiodarone, ASA, quinidine, quinine
    O ral neomycin
    U rokinase and streptokinase
    M iconazole
    A ntibiotics (*CHEMIST*: **Ch**loramphenicol, **E**rythromycin, **M**etronidazole, **I**soniazid, **S**ulfonamides, **TC**N)
    D iuretics: thiazides and ethacrynic acid
    I nfluenza vaccine
    N SAIDs

    P henylbutazone, Propylthiouracil, propoxyphene
    A cute alcohol use, allopurinol, anabolic steroids, antabuse
    C hloral hydrate, cimetidine, clofibrate
    T hyroxine

Meds that Decrease Warfarin Level: *DECREASE*:

    D iuretics: spironolactone
    E strogen-containing OCPs
    C arbamazepine, corticosteroids
    R ifampin
    E thylchlorvynol
    S ucralfate
    E tc: barbiturates, griseofulvin, and vit K

LOW MOLECULAR-WEIGHT Heparin- - ADVANTAGES Over Conventional Heparin:

1. *Precludes daily PTT* determination
2. *More predictable* response
3. *Better safety* profile
4. Ease of administration
5. And, of course, less time in the hospital

OUTPATIENT DVT MANAGEMENT with Enoxaparin (a Low Molecular Weight Heparin):

1. If patient is appropriate for outpatient therapy[1] , arrange instruction in self-injection thru a home health nurse.
2. Educate about the side effects of LMWH and signs/symptoms of a PE
3. Dosing of enoxaparin is **1mg/kg SC q 12h**
4. **Start warfarin, 5-10 mg/d on day 1 or 2 of enoxaparin**
5. √ a CBC with platelets after 5-7 days of enoxaparin. Check the INR every 2-3 days after starting warfarin.
6. **Continue LMWH until the INR is between 2.0-3.0**
7. **Continue warfarin for 3-6 months**, but consider long-term treatment with warfarin if this is a 2nd episode of DVT.

[1] *Patient should not have any of the following*:
   a. Active PUD
   b. Concurrent symptomatic PE
   c. Current active bleeding
   d. Familial bleeding disorder
   e. Inability to use LMWH because of some coexistant disease
   f. Known deficiency of AT III, Protein C, or Protein S
   g. Noncompliance
   h. Pregnancy
   i. ≥ 2 prior episodes of DVT or PE

DVT PROPHYLAXIS	
PATIENT POPULATION	**RECOMMENDED PROPHYLAXIS**
Low-risk general surgery patients	Early ambulation
Moderate-risk general surgery patients	LDUH (low-dose unfractionated heparin), LMWH (low molecular weight heparin), intermittent pneumatic compression (IPC), elastic stockings (ES)
High-risk general surgery patients	LDUH or higher-dosage LMWH
Higher-risk general surgery patients prone to wound complications	IPC is an alternative
Very-high-risk general surgery patients with multiple risk factors	LDUH or LMWH, combined with IPC
Selected very-high-risk general surgery patients	Perioperative warfarin (goal INR 2-3)
Patients undergoing THR	LMWH, started 12-24h postop; or warfarin, started before or immediately after surgery or adjusted-dose heparin, started preoperatively; possible adjuvant use of ES or IPC
Patients undergoing TKR	LMWH, warfarin, or IPC
Patients undergoing hip fracture surgery	LMWH, or warfarin started preop or immediately postop
High-risk patients undergoing orthopedic surgery	IVC filter placement only when anticoagulant-based prophylaxis is not feasible because of active bleeding

Patients undergoing intracranial surgery	IPC ± ES; LMWH and LDUH may be acceptable alternatives; consider IPC or ES + LMWH or LDUH for high-risk patients
Patients with MI	LDUH or full-dose anticoagulation; IPC and possible ES may be useful when heparin is contraindicated
Patients with ischemic CVA and lower extrem. paralysis	LDUH or LMWH; IPC with ES also is probably effective
General medical patients with clinical risk factors for DVT, particularly those with CHF or chest infections	LDUH or LMWH
Patients with long-term indwelling central vein catheters	Warfarin, 1mg/d, or LMWH, qd, to prevent axillary-subclavian venous thrombosis
Patients having spinal puncture or epidural catheters placed for regional anesthesia or analgesia	LMWH should be used with caution

Abbreviations
- LDUH =low-dose unfractionated heparin
- LMWH =low molecular weight heparin
- IPC=intermittent pneumatic compression
- ES=Elastic stockings
- THR=Total hip replacement
- TKR=Total knee replacement

APLASTIC ANEMIA

1. 2° to a stem cell defect

2. **Pancytopenia**, hypocellular bone marrow

3. **Mortality 80% at 2 years unless allo BMT or ATG (antithymocyte globulin)**

4. Idiopathic is #1 cause

5. Drugs are #2 cause

6. **PNH and infections (Hepatitis B and C)** ✪ are #3 cause.

7. **Take special care with transfusions!** If transfusions are needed, select nonrelated donors and use leuk-depleted PRBCs and single-donor platelets. Family members should not be transfusion donors since they are more likely to sensitize the patient to minor HLA antigens present in the donor, but absent in the patient.

8. BMT carries a 65% success rate in young patients

9. If older than 45-50 and no HLA match→treatment is ATG instead

ITP (Idiopathic Thrombocytopenic Purpura)

- **Drugs commonly implicated**→procainamide; quinine; quinidine; heparin; gold; sulfonamides; and rifampin.

- *Treatment* ✪
    1. *Steroids*—the mainstay of treatment; used first to decrease Ab production
    2. If #1 fails →*splenectomy* to remove the predominant site of Ab production and platelet destruction.
    3. If #2 fails→ *chemotherapy*

- *Note these mechanisms of action:*

    1) High dose gamma globulin **BLOCKS the Fc receptors** of phagocytic cells and is used in emergency bleeding only.

    2) Danazol works by ↓ **the NUMBER** of phagocytic cell Fc receptors.

HEMOCHROMATOSIS (Systemic Disease Of Iron Overload)

1. *Remember*: transferrin sat>62% in men and > 50% in women—best SCREENING test.

2. **Clinical:**
    a. **Endocrine**
        i. DM
        ii. Hypogonadism (impotence, libido, amenorrhea)↓
        iii. Hypopituitarism
    b. **Liver**
        i. Hepatomegaly
        ii. Cirrhosis (can lead to hepatocellular carcinoma)
    c. **Skin**
        i. Bronze ("bronze diabetes")
    d. **Cardiac**
        i. CHF
        ii. Arrythmias
    e. **Arthropathy**

3. **IRREVERSIBLE COMPLICATIONS** ✪ in hemochromatosis:
    a. *Arthropathy*
    b. *Hypogonadism*
    c. HCC (Hepatocellular carcinoma)
    d. Hepatic cirrhosis

APPENDIX

Figure 1.   <u>**Hemolytic Anemia:**</u>

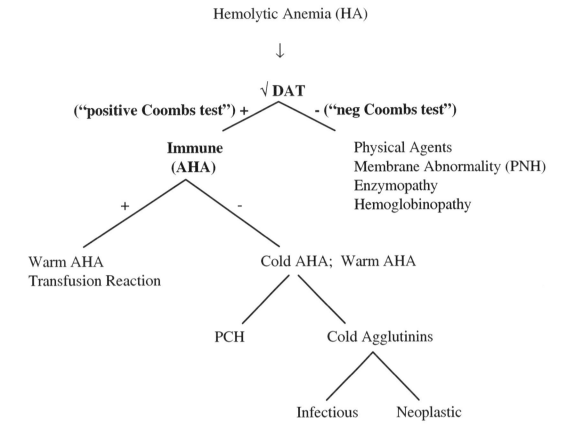

Figure 2   <u>**Approach to Thrombocytopenia:**</u>

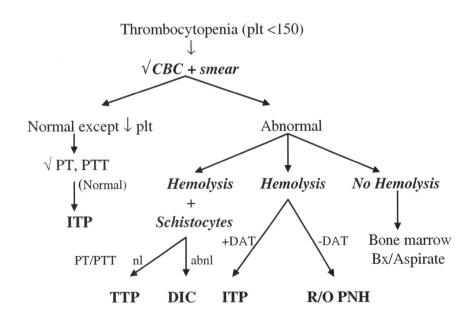

Figure 3.   <u>**Overview to the Intrinsic & Extrinsic Clotting Cascade:**</u>

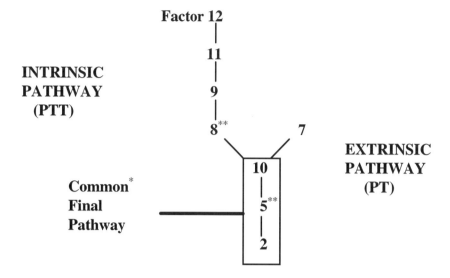

*Remember: $\uparrow$ PT or PTT may also be 2° to deficiencies in factors of the common final pathway.

**Remember too: Protein C(with the help of cofactor Protein S) work to degrade factors 8 and 5; thus deficiencies in these proteins confer a *hyper*coaguable state.

<u>A breakdown of the final steps of the coagulation cascade shows</u>:

♦ **Factor 10 + 5 take Prothrombin → Thrombin, which in turn takes Fibrinogen → Fibrin.**

♦ **Then Factor 13 helps to cross-link the fibrin monomers.**

2. ONCOLOGY

BREAST CA

Who's at risk?
1. Previous h/o breast ca
2. Family history of breast ca
3. early menarche, late first pregnancy, or late menopause—all situations of prolonged estrogen exposure
4. Radiation Exposure at an early age
5. "Benign" breast disease in the form of atypical ductal hyperplasia
6. OCPs and postmenopausal HRT 2° to Estrogen

Speaking of HRT...
   ✪ **Facts you should know about Evista® (Raloxifene):**
   ⇒ a SERM (Selective Estrogen Receptor Modulator)
   ⇒ Indicated for prevention of osteoporosis in postmenopausal women;
   ⇒ ↓ risk of breast ca (hormone receptor positive breast ca)
   ⇒ *No* ↑ risk of uterine ca
   ⇒ Does *not* control perimenopausal symptoms, such as hot flashes.

How do you screen?
1. Monthly self breast exams
2. Annual clinical breast exam ≥ 40 yo
3. Annual mammogram, now acceptable ≥ 40 yo as well

Primary Treatment of Breast Ca
- Either: a) *MRM* (modified radical mastectomy) + ALND (axillary lymph node dissection) followed by ± XRT (radiation) or b) *lumpectomy* + ALND definitely followed by XRT

Adjuvant Systemic Therapy
- *Depends on these 3 factors:*
   i. Pre or Postmenopausal   *and*
   ii. ER + or -   *and*
   iii. Lymph node status (axillary)

Here's how it works...

If Lymph Nodes + or LN -

	ER +	ER -
Premenopausal	Chemo *(or Tamox if LN neg)*	Chemo
Postmenopausal	Tamoxifen	Consider Chemo

✪ CRITICAL GENERAL CONCEPTS IN BREAST CA:

1. The breakdown of breast carcinoma:
   - 80% are infiltrating (or "invasive") ductal
   - 10% are infiltrating lobular
     - Remember, there is a 50% incidence of *bilaterality* in lobular breast ca
   - The prognosis is similar for infiltrating ductal and infiltrating lobular
   - Medullary and a few others constitute the rest

2. Axillary dissection is needed for *all* patients, whether MRM **or** lumpectomy.

3. If given a breast ca patient with 1 or more *positive <u>Supraclavicular</u> lymph node(s)* on her physical exam, that's automatically <u>Stage 4</u>!

4. *XRT is not routinely indicated/not necessarily indicated following the lymph node dissection of a MRM* and can unnecessarily result in lymphedema, as opposed to lymph node dissection + lumpectomy, where XRT is always indicated.

5. *Node positive premenopausal* patients get chemo *no matter* what their ER status.

6. *Most patients with node negative disease are cured with primary* treatment alone (i.e. without adjuvant/systemic therapy); adjuvant therapy however offers greater assurance with improved cure rates.

7. In fact, *unless* the patient has *unfavorable tumor features* [high mitotic activity (high S phase), large tumor (> 2.5cm) (another poor feature), undifferentiated/poorly differentiated histology, tumor adherent to skin, chest wall, or pectoralis muscle, matty lymph nodes or + SC nodes, and Her2neu receptor status], **node negative patients with tumors ≤ 1 cm should not receive adjuvant therapy**.

8. In *metastatic ER+* disease, oophorectomy (for premenopausal) or hormonal therapy (for postmenopausal) if there is no visceral involvement.

9. If *metastatic ER -* disease with visceral involvement→CMF or CAF chemo

10. Recall that of all the *prognosticators* in breast ca, positive *lymph nodes* is the most reliable.

11. Remember that *Inflammatory Breast Ca*
    - Requires a biopsy to differentiate it from cellulitis or mastitis;
    - It involves rapid progression of skin edema, ridging, and diffuse erythema.
    - Requires aggressive chemotherapy

CERVICAL CA

- Pap smears are critical in screening for this carcinoma.

- *HPV* (Human Papilloma Virus), considered an STD, is the causative agent and, understandably, is rarely, if ever, found in celebate nuns.

- *HSV II* has also been found to be associated with this cancer.

- Screening is recommended with Pap smears as follows
    1. *Yearly at onset of sexual activity or starting at age 18*
    2. *Every 1-3 years after 3 consecutive smears are negative*

COLON CA

Remember...

1. Most tumors start as adenomatous polyps, and the *progression* is from normal mucosa→polyp→cancer over 10 years. Therefore, the risk of a polyp becoming cancerous is related to both size and time. ✪

2. Clinically significant polyps are those measuring > *7mm* (just over ½ cm). ✪

3. After lung, colon ca is the 2nd leading cause of cancer death. ✪

4. After patient's have *Ulcerative Colitis* for 30 years, they have a 1 in 2 chance of developing colon cancer; periodic biopsies should therefore be taken to check for dysplasia, which necessitates colectomy.

5. One's risk of developing colorectal ca is *2-3x* ↑ *if a first degree relative* has had this carcinoma.

6. *Personal h/o breast, uterine, or ovarian ca doubles your risk.*

7. 100% of patients with *FAP* have become malignant by age 40yo
    a) Screening in affected families: colonoscopy Qyear ≥puberty.
    b) EGD Q 3-5 years after polyps are the first polyps are found.

8. *High fat, low fiber diets* are associated with colorectal ca.

9. In *Peutz-Jeghers syndrome, as opposed to Gardner's syndrome*, the polyps are benign and are not at significant ↑ risk of malignant transformation than regular adenomatous polyps.

10. Recall that polyps are either hyperplastic or adenomatous. Hyperplastic polyps do not have malignant potential. Know that between *tubular* polyps and *villous* polyps, while tubular are much more common, villous polyps are the true "villains" in their malignant potential.

SCREENING—_See GI for new ACS criteria on colorectal carcinoma screening/polyp surveillance._

DUKE'S CLASSIFICATION FOR COLORECTAL CA:

Stage	Definition	Treatment
A	Confined to mucosa/submucosa	Surgery
B1	Muscularis mucosa	Surgery
B2	*thru SEROSA*	Surg + Chemo
	(**Remember**, when it comes to the boards, one can never "B2 SERious"…)	
C1	+ regional lymph node mets ≤4	Surg + Chemo
C2	+ regional lymph node mets >4	Surg + Chemo
D	Distant mets	Surg + Chemo

- *CEA* is not for screening! Only use it for follow-up only to check for recurrence.

- **5FU (5-fluorouracil) and levamisole** is the Adjuvant Therapy used for Stages ≥ B

RECTAL CA
* **5FU and XRT** is the Adjuvant Treatment

CHEMO-RELATED TOXICITIES FOR THE BOARDS

Adriamycin (Doxorubicin)→dose-related cardiomyopathy and CHF

Bleomycin, **B**CNU (Carmustine), **B**usulfan→ all can give Pulmonary fibrosis. Remember fibrosis is tough, so remember on the boards→"***B tough***!"

Cisplatin→
1. Peripheral neuropathy (similar to Vincristine);
2. Renal tubular damage;
3. Tinnitus & hearing loss.

Cyclophosphamide→
1. Bone: Myelosuppression (see also Melphalan)
2. Bladder: Hemorrhagic cystitis; bladder ca (see also Melphalan)
3. GU: Sterility in males; amenorrhea.

5FU→
1. Mucositis
2. Cerebellar ataxia

Melphalan→
1. Bone: Myelosuppression
2. Bladder: Hemorrhagic cystitis; bladder ca
3. Leukemia

Methotrexate→
1. Renal toxicity
2. Pulmonary fibrosis (see also Bleomycin)
3. Postnecrotic cirrhosis

Mitomycin C → <u>HUS</u> (*Hemolytic Uremic Syndrome*)

Tamoxifen (non-chemo adjuvant tx)→
1. Thrombophlebitis
2. ↑ risk of uterine ca
3. ↓ risk of cardiac disease
4. Bone pain, vaginal dryness, hot flashes

Taxol → Cardiac toxicity

Vincristine → Peripheral neuropathy

POTENTIALLY CURABLE CANCERS FOR THE BOARDS
1. Ewings sarcoma
2. Hodgkin's and NHL
3. Leukemias, acute and chronic
4. Testicular ca

ESOPHAGEAL CA (SCC)

Risk factors:
1. *Alcohol*
2. *Tobacco*
3. *Barrett's esophagus*/ Barrett's esophagus with dysplasia
4. Plummer-Vinson syndrome
5. Ingestion of…
   a) Smoked or pickled foods
   b) Lye
6. *Achalasia*
7. Tylosis

HEPATOCELLULAR CA (HCC, "Hepatoma")
1. Any cirrhosis ↑s the risk of HCC, but especially…
   a) HBV, HBC
   b) Alcoholic liver disease
   c) Hemochromatosis
2. Half the time ***alpha-fetoprotein*** is ↑.
3. Resection is the treatment of choice, as transplantation is complicated by a high rate of recurrence.

LUNG CA

- *Screening is not warranted* in lung ca, as opposed to cervical, breast, and colon carcinomas, so "annual chest x-rays" is not appropriate in a preventitive care visit of a low-risk/no-risk non-smoker. In smokers over 50, annual CXR is useful in detecting Stage I disease.

- The main types are **small** cell (also known as oat cell); **squamous** cell; **large** cell; and **adeno** ca. The first 2 are central, and the last two are peripherally located. All four are associated with smoking. Broncho-alveolar lung ca (rare) is not.

    - ✪ Remember, **SMALL** cell and **SQUAMOUS** cell ca lung ca are *Sentral* (centrally located).
    - ✪ Remember too, just as **LARGE** cell and **ADENO** ca are peripheral, so either can result in *"peripheral"* findings as seen at the finger tips! (Hypertrophic Osteoarthopathy, HOA)

- Remember, *Adenoca*, the other primary peripheral ca, is the most common of these four types among non-smokers; it is also known as *"scar carcinoma"*.

- **POTENTIAL COMPLICATIONS** of the four types you must know for the boards:

    - ✪ *Squamous*→ May Cavitate; ↑ Calcium (ectopic production of **PTH**-like hormone; Sympathetic nerve paralysis ("Horner's syndrome": miosis; **P**tosis; anhydrosis); **P**ancoast's tumor (with growth into the brachial plexus, C8-T2).

    - ✪ *Small cell*→ "AACES":

        ↑ADH (SIADH)

        ↑ACTH (Cushing's syndrome)

        Carcinoid

        Eaton-Lambert Syndrome
        - Muscle weakness, noted in simple tasks like combing one's hair or rising from a chair
        - Improves with effort/repetitive action

        SVC

        ┌───┐
        │ ♦ Remember the commonly quoted fact in small cell: "The #1 cause of death in survivors of small cell lung ca is *non-small* cell lung ca!" │
        └───┘

- *Large cell and adeno ca*→ HOA (as noted above)

STAGING AND TREATMENT

- *For treatment purposes, in lung ca the carcinomas are divided into either…*
    1. **Small cell; or**
    2. **Non-small cell**

    …because *staging and managment differ* between small cell and all the others.

- ✪ Because **Small cell** ca is usually fairly advanced at the time of diagnosis, ***Chemo and XRT*** are the treatments of choice, **as opposed to Non-small cell,** where *Surgery* is the treatment of choice in the early stages (I-IIIA).

Mediastinoscopy/otomy very important in staging; "oscopy" for the right side (no obstruction from the heart, so easier to look around); "otomy" for the left.

- Because of this key difference in mangagement, *staging is viewed slighlty differently* for small cell and non-small cell and goes as follows:

NON-SMALL CELL Lung Ca ✪

Stage	*Criteria*	*Treatment*
I	- Hilar nodes	**SURGERY**
II	+ Hilar nodes	**SURGERY**
III A	**IPSILATERAL** involvement of the MED/SC nodes or CW	**SURGERY**
III **B**	Goes ***CONTRALATERAL*** *(REMEMBER, "B" for "Bilateral")*	Chemo+XRT ✪
IV	Distant Disease (as always)	Chemo+XRT

SMALL CELL Lung Ca ✪

"Limited Disease" = Stages I-IIIA	→	**Chemo+XRT**
vs.		
"Extensive Disease"= Metastases	→	**Chemo only**

Beyond staging, there are additional criteria for operative candidate:

1. **Lung lesion > 2cm from carina**

2. **Involvement of no major vessels**

3. **If preop FEV1 < 2L, MVV <50%, or DLCO <60%, need a quantitative V/Q scan to assess the expected post-op FEV1, which must be >1.3L**

4. **Resting pCO2 >50**

   - *Severe COPD and pCO2 >45-50 going into the surgery are considered negative prognosticators.*

HODGKIN'S LYMPHOMA

1. See **Reed-Sternberg cells** on pathology

2. 50% have **EBV** genome incorporated into their DNA

3. Remember, staging in HL is based on **location** of tumor relative to diaphragm, as opposed to staging in NHL, which is based on **histology** (cell type), as specific cell types are classified differently (Low grade; Intermediate grade; High grade; Misc) depending on their aggressiveness and treatment, as seen here...

STAGE	CRITERIA	TREATMENT
I	One LN region, one side of diaphragm	**XRT**
II	Two LN regions, one side of diaphragm	**XRT**
IIIA1	Both sides of diaphragm have + LN	**XRT**
---	---	---
IIIA2	IIIA1 with additional LN sets involved	Chemo
	(Why "A2" and not "B"? You don't want to confuse with "b symptoms", which one can have at any stage and may include fever, night sweats, weight loss)	
IV	Disseminated disease (bone marrow; liver)	Chemo

- ✪ Note: **Treatment of Stages I-IIIA₁ is XRT !!**

- ✪ You must make sure all *apparent "Stage I and II's" are not actually III's → must do staging laparotomy since may not need chemo!*

- ✪ Remember, *in Stages II and III,* **add Chemo** *(to XRT)* **if "bulky disease"** (the exception).

- *Chemo is **ABVD** (less toxic than MOPP); **CHOP** is used for NHL.*

•*Those who survive the initial chemo may SECONDARILY develop:*
1. **AML**

2. **Solid tumors**;

3. **Diffuse, aggressive lymphomas**.

NON-HODGKIN'S (NHL):

<u>**Low grades**</u> (*these have <u>long survival times and at most stages are very responsive to initial therapy, but are not curable</u> and include…*)

   1. Multiple Myeloma

   2. Waldenstrom's Macroglobulinemia

   3. CLL

<u>**Intermediate Grades**</u> (*<u>curable, but poor survival if don't survive initial chemo—re: CHOP</u>*)

   • *DLCL* (Diffuse Large Cell Lymphoma) falls under here

<u>**High Grades**</u> (*also may be curable*)

   1. Lymphoblastic lymphoma (a T-cell lymphoma; may goto CNS and bone marrow); chemo similar to ALL

   2. Small non-cleaved

      (a) *Burkitt's* (EBV causes)

         (i) American subtype—intraabdominal tumor→bone and CNS
         (ii) African subset—jaw tumor

      (b) *Non-Burkitt's*

<u>**Miscellaneous**</u>

   • *Mycosis Fungoides* falls here.

Important Reminders...

- Remember, *serum LDH* can be very useful in estimating the aggressiveness and actual spread of an NHL

- *Staging laparotomy is not common in NHL*, since chemo is usually the treatment of choice and spread of NHL is generally hematogenous, as opposed to contiguous (from 1 set of nodes to the next)

- Since *low grades* usually present late stage, observation is the rule, since not cured with chemo.

- If *high grades* initially completely responds to chemo, but then relapse, consider BMT.

MALIGNANCIES ASSOCIATED WITH AIDS

1. HL and NHL as well as CNS Lymphoma
2. Cervical ca
3. Kaposi's sarcoma
4. Anal carcinoma

MULTIPLE MYELOMA ✪

- **M-protein is > 3g/dl**

- **Plasma cells in the bone marrow > 10%**

- **Urinary light chains (Bence Jones proteins)**

- **Anemia** (normocytic, normochromic)—check for *Rouleau* formation on the PBS; ↑ Ca; ↑ **creat; osteolytic** (*"punched out"*)bone lesions 2° to **OAF** (osteoclast-activating factor)—invisible on bone scan since no new bone formation occurs. See osteolytic vs. osteoblastic section below.

- **Clinically** in order (most common to least common): bone pain; renal insufficiency; hypercalcemia; weakness, fatigue, and spinal cord compression

- ↑**Incidence:**
    i. Pneumococcal pneumonia
    ii. Gram-negative infections
    iii. Herpes Zoster

- *Melphalan and Prednisone* commonly used in the *treatment* of this incurable disease. Treatment should be **delayed** until *either* evidence of progression or imminent complications.

MONOCLONAL GAMMOPATHY ✪ (MGUS is abbrev for "monoclonal gammopathy of undetermined significance")

- **M-protein is < 3g/dl**

- **plasma cells in the bone marrow < 10%**

- No anemia or osteolytic bone lesions, as opposed to MM

- 20% become malignant

OSTEOLYTIC *versus* OSTEOBLASTIC LESIONS

> - **Purely osteolytic lesions → MM and renal cell ca**
> - Osteoblastic lesions → prostate and breast ca

PANCREATIC CA

- The primary etiology in "*adenoca of unknown primary*", so when you don't know what the source of the adenoca metastasis is, check either CT or U/S of the pancreas.

- Remember that even before patient's are told they have pancreatic ca and even before they are symptomatic, there is an ↑ risk of pancreatic ca having an endogenous *depression*, which is felt to be 2° to an unknown paraneoplastic substrate.

- ↑ incidence of *migratory thrombophlebitis* (so called "Trouseau's Syndrome"✪)

PROSTATE CA

- *The ACS (American Cancer Society) recommends DRE Q year >40 and PSA Q year > 50. Discontinue when life expectancy< 10 years.*

- *PSA values: <4 is OK; 4-10 is observation and/or TRUS (Transrectal U/S) ± biopsy; >10 should undergo TRUS + biopsy*

- *30-40% of men>60 have malignant prostate cells and will die WITH them, not OF them.* Only 8-9% of these individuals will be diagnosed with prostate ca per se. And only a small % of those will die OF prostate ca. Remember, growth into a clinically important ca takes up to 15 years. It's all about the quality and quantity (if any) of years that you're adding by screening and follow-up compared to the side-effects the treatment will cause. These side effects may include: impotence (usually from the XRT or prostatectomy). That's the controversy!

- **Significance of % Free PSA:**

  - Useful in eliminating unnecessary prostate biopsies in the diagnostic "gray zone" (PSA 4-10). A *low total % free PSA* (<25%) is associated with ↑ risk of malignancy.
  - % free PSA has no role in the initial evaluation of men with an abnormal DRE, as they should all proceed to biopsy.
  - For total PSA in the range of 4-10 ng/mL, % free PSA should be measured. If <25% → prostate biopsy. If ≥ 25% → annual total PSA and DRE. Cutoff at this level of 25% eliminates 20% of unnecessary biopsies with resulting sensitivity of 95%.

- The men at ↑**risk** are those African-Americans and those with + Fam Hx.

Risk factor:	*Risk of developing prostate ca:*
A frican-American	2x the relative risk
F ather had it	3x the relative risk
B rother had it	4x the relative risk

Remember "A→F→B" for the order of which is 2, which is 3, and which is 4.

- As with breast ca, this is a hormonally-driven ca, by androgens, no estrogen.

STAGING & TREATMENT

Stage	Criteria	Treatment
A1	*Microscopic*; <5% of specimen	Observation
A2	*Microscopic*; >5% of specimen	**Prostatectomy versus XRT**
B1	**1 *nodule*, limited to 1 lobe**	" " "
B2	**Several *nodules*, both lobes**	" " "
C	**C**apsular &/or Extra**C**apsular (e.g. the seminal vesicles)	XRT/radioactive seed implant
D1	Pelvic nodes +	(controversial)
D2	Distant mets	Androgen deprivation

Staging & Treatment of Prostate Ca cont'd...

- Results of *XRT and prostatectomy* are comparable, and XRT is less likely to cause impotence than prostatectomy

- Results of *anti-androgen therapy and orchiectomy* are comparable for Stage D2

- *Total androgen ablation* is usually achieved using **leuprolide** (Leupron®), actually an LHRH agonist which acts to ultimately inhibit androgen production, plus **flutamide** (Eulexin®), which inhibits androgen binding to its receptor. Remember too that androgens are also produced in the adrenal cortex, and this can be stopped too using **aminoglutethimide**.

- *Implantable radioactive seeds* are rapidly gaining acceptance, at least as an additional therapeutic alternative to XRT and even prostatectomy.

SKIN CA

1. *SQUAMOUS CELL CA—re: actinic keratosis is premalignant for SCC*

2. *MALIGNANT MELANOMA*

   i) Similar to breast ca, the *incidence* of malignant melanoma is ↑ing rapidly 2° to earlier dx

   ii) Know the *risk factors*...

      a) Repeated and/or blistering sun exposure as a child
      b) + FH
      c) Fair skin
      d) Dysplastic nevi—the source of half of melanomas

   iii) Obviously must know, *ABCD* keys to diagnosis: Asymmetry; Borders irregular; Color is variable, esp with blues/blacks/tans; Diameter ≥ 6mm

   iv) ✪ *Not to be confused with the above 6mm (!), you should know that the best independent predictor of survival is the thickness of the melanoma on biopsy, and that thickness you hope is ≤.76mm for high chance of survival.*

   v) Re: *Moh's surgery* ✪ is both diagnostic and therapeutic and involves essentially shaving off the lesion tier by tier until the margins are clear per the pathologist. Melanoma is not the only indication for Moh's surgery, which can be used in tumors involving cosmetically or aesthetically sensitive zones.

   vi) Remember *sentinel lymph node mapping* ✪ is used for melanoma and is increasingly being used for breast ca (to spare the patient unnecessarily extensive lymph node dissections)

SKIN DISEASE AS MANIFESTATION OF MALIGNANCY

1. Acanthosis nigricans (not just DM and obesity!)→GI malignancy, esp gastric; also most conditions associated with insulin resistance. See Dermatology for more on acanthosis nigricans.
2. Actinic keratosis→SCC
3. Café au lait spots→ Von Recklinghausen's disease
4. Dysplastic nevus→Malignant melanoma
5. Epidermal cysts, fibromas, lipomas→Gardner's syndrome
6. Flushing, telangiectasias→Carcinoid tumors
7. Mucosal hyperpigmentation (esp. lips)→ Peutz-Jeghers syndrome
8. Necrolytic erythematous rash (NME: Necrolytic Migratory Erythema)→Glucagonoma

IMPORTANT POINTS ON BRCA1 AND BRCA2:

- ↑ Risk of breast and ovarian ca
- **BRCA 1 & 2 are tumor suppression genes. Mutations to these genes "unsuppresses" ca risk** and confers an ↑d risk of ca in an autosomal dominant fashion; 5-10% of all cases of breast ca
- The cumulative risk (to age 70) of developing **breast ca in females** due to mutations of either BRCA 1 or 2 is 60-80%, vs. cumulative 11% risk in the population at large (up to age 79)
- Also, while there is a significant ↑ in relative risk (6% vs. .1% for population at large) of developing **breast ca in males** with BRCA2 mutation, there is no ↑d relative risk in men who have BRCA1.
- By age 70, women with BRCA1 mutations also have an **ovarian cancer** risk of up to 40% (20% for BRCA2).
- **Genetic testing is indicated** only if the prior probability of abnormalities is ≥ 10%, as revealed by family and clinical history. But in general, testing would be appropriate in each of the following situations:
    1. Patient has ≥ 2 blood relatives—mother, sister, aunt, cousin, or daughter—with premenopausal breast ca or ovarian ca at any age;
    2. Patient has been diagnosed with breast ca, esp premenopause, *and* has a blood relative w/ breast or ovarian cancer;
    3. Patient with ≥ 2 family members with breast cancer diagnosed < 50 yo
    4. Patient has been diagnosed with ovarian ca and has blood relatives who have had ovarian c breast ca;
    5. Patient is related to someone (male or female) who has a BRCA 1 or 2 mutation.
    6. Male patient with breast cancer
    7. Early-onset (<50 yo) breast or ovarian ca in patients of Ashkenazi Jewish ancestry.
- Patients found to carry these mutations should be encouraged to commit to an intensive, lifelong program of cancer surveillance.

- **Women with a BRCA mutation should have a:**
    ⇒ Mammogram every year beginning at age 25 yo
    ⇒ Clinical breast exam 1-2 times/y beginning at 25 yo
    ⇒ BSE q mo > 18 yo
    ⇒ A pelvic exam once or twice a year beginning at 25-35yo
    ⇒ Transvaginal U/S with color doppler once or twice a year starting at 25-35 yo
    ⇒ Serum CA 125 every year beginning age 25-35 yo.

REVISED CRITERIA FOR THE DX OF HNPCC (Hereditary Nonpolyposis Colorectal Cancer)

*   *≥ 3 relatives with an HNPCC-associated cancer* (colon, endometrium, ovary, small bowel, ureter, renal pelvis)
    *   ≥ 1 should be a 1st degree relative of the other 2
    *   ≥ 2 successive generations affected
    *   ≥ 1 relative diagnosed before age 50

*   *Tumor should be assessed pathologically*

*   *FAP should be excluded*

TESTICULAR CA

Basics first...

1. The #1 ca in males 15-35 yo

2. The biggest risk factor is ***cryptorchidism***, or undescended testes. ***Surgically bringing down the teste does not reduce the risk of ca.*** Klinefelter's is another risk factor.

3. Similar to lung ca or Hodgkins, there are 2 overall categories...
    a)   Seminomas
    b)   Non-seminomas

4. **SEM**inomas are highly radio**SEN**sitive, and only 10% secrete Beta-HCG; never AFP!!

5. **Non-seminomas** on the other hand do not respond to XRT and secrete both AFP and Beta-HCG. This is clearly summarized in the following table ✪:

	SEMINOMA	NON-SEMINOMA
AFP	**No**	Yes
B-HCG	Yes	Yes

6. ✪   The primary ***treatment*** is radical (inguinal) orchiectomy. Then, if the biopsy shows seminoma, the treatment is **XRT** for Stages 1 and 2. For Stage 1 non-seminoma, surgery followed by observation is usually sufficient. ***For everything else***, it's **platinum-based** chemo! Study the following...

See next page for staging & treatment...

STAGE	CRITERIA	SEMINOMA	vs.	NONSEMINOMA
I	Limited to testes	Surg→**XRT**		Surg→observe
II	→ Peritoneum (low grade: < 6LN+ and LN < 2cm)	**XRT**		Chemo
III	→ Peritoneum (high grade: >6LN+ or LN > 2cm)	Chemo		Chemo
IV	Distant mets	Chemo		Chemo

7. ✪ Remember, *testicular carcinoma is <u>highly curable, even when metastatic</u>* (e.g. to the mediastinum).

8. ✪ Finally, remember that if any solitary *lung mets* are detected post-chemo, they may be surgically *removed*.

3. **CANCER STAGING & TREATMENT SIMPLIFIED**

The Nomenclature of Staging:

"1234s"

Small Cell/ NSC
Hodgkins/ NHL
Seminoma/Nonseminoma
Breast Carcinoma

"ABCDs"

Colon Ca.
Prostate Ca.

ABCD's

Colon Carcinoma

		Treatment
A	mucosa/submucosa	$S_{(urg)}$
B_1	muscularis	"

B_2	thru *serosa*	$S+C_{(hemo)}$
C	+ LNs	"
D	istant	"

Prostate Carcinoma

A_1	< 5% specimen	Observe
A_2	> 5% specimen	S vs $X_{(RT)}$
B_1	1 lobe/1 nodule	"
B_2	2 lobes/≥ 2 nodules	"

C	apsular/Extracapsular	X/implantable seeds
D	istant	Androgen Ablation

1234's

Non-Small Cell Lung Ca

1	Hilar LN -	S
2	Hilar LN +	S
3A	*Ipsilat.* med/SC LN or CW+	S

3B	*Contralat.* " " " " "	C+X
4	Distant	C+X

Small Cell Lung Ca

1-3A	"Limited Disease"	C+X
3B,4	"Extensive Disease"	C

Hodgkin's Lymphoma (Ann Arbor Criteria)

1	1set of LN, 1 side diaphragm	X
2	>1 set " " " " "	X
3A$_1$	Both sides diaphragm, *upper* abd.	X

3A$_2$	Both sides diaphragm, *lower* abd.	C
4	Distant	C

Testicular Ca

		Sem	Non-Sem
1	Testes only	S→X	S→Observe
2	Peritoneal LN (<6; <2cm)	X	C
3	Peritoneal LN (>6; >2cm)	C	C
4	Distant	C	C

Breast Ca   (Stages 0-4)

0	Carcinoma in situ (intraductal or lobular); 5y survival >95%
1	1° tumor<2cm, neg axillary LNs; 5y survival 85%
2A	1° tumor <2cm & +ax LNs *or* 2-5cm & -LNs; 5y survival 75%
2B	1° tumor 2-5cm & + ax LNs *or* >5cm & - LNs; 5y survival 65%
3A	Tumor> 5cm & + ipsilateral ax LNs or fixed LNs; 5y=50%
3B	Involvement of IM LNs/Chest wall/ulcerated skin; 5y=41%
4	Distant mets; 5y survival 10%

Stage III Breast Ca

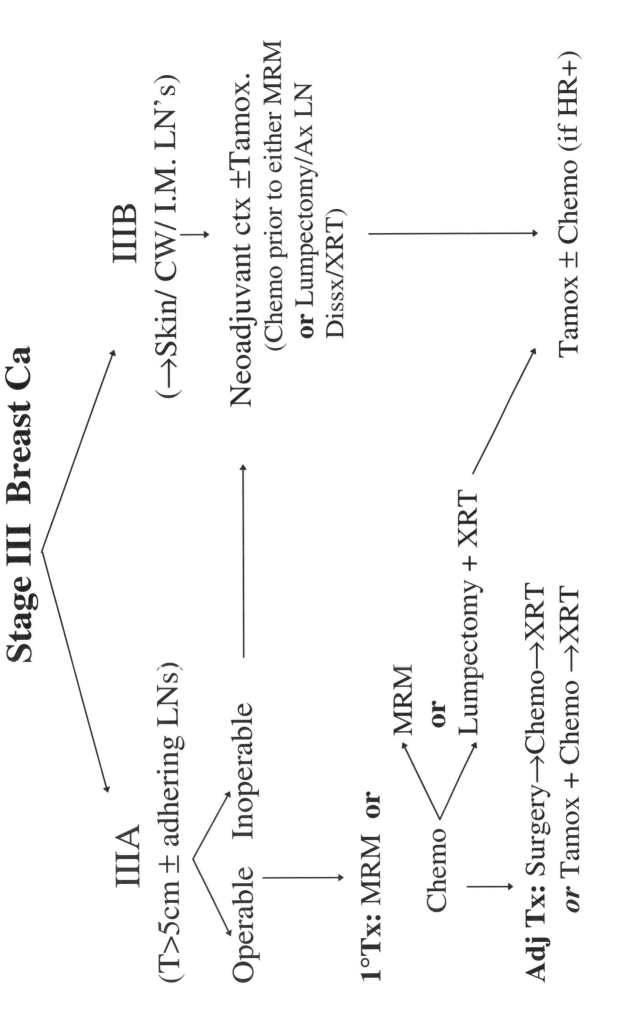

IIIA

(T>5cm ± adhering LNs)

Operable   Inoperable

1°Tx: MRM or

Chemo

MRM
or
Lumpectomy + XRT

Adj Tx: Surgery→Chemo→XRT
or Tamox + Chemo →XRT

IIIB

(→Skin/ CW/ I.M. LN's)

Neoadjuvant ctx ±Tamox.

(Chemo prior to either MRM
or Lumpectomy/Ax LN
Dissx/XRT)

Tamox ± Chemo (if HR+)

Stage IV Breast Ca

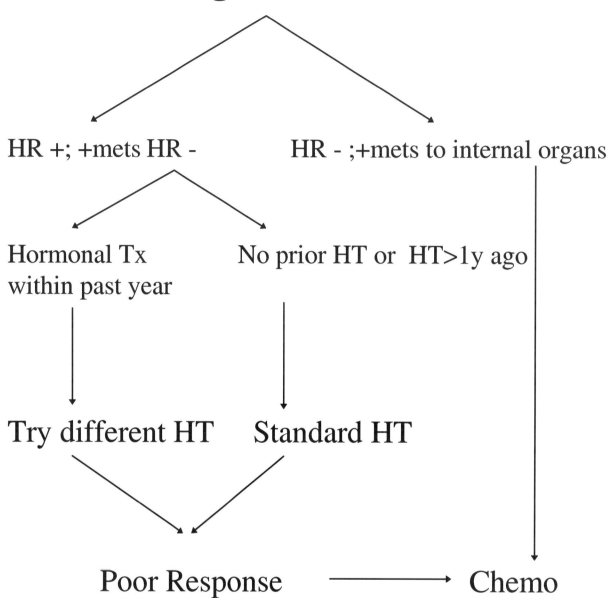

4. <u>RHEUMATOLOGY</u>

Seven Diagnostic Criteria for Rheumatoid Arthritis*
1. Morning stiffness
2. Arthritis of ≥ 3 joint areas
3. Arthritis of the hand joints
4. Symmetric arthritis
5. Rheumatoid nodules
6. Serum rheumatoid factor
7. Radiographic changes

> * In order to have RA, you must have ≥4 of the 7 criteria present and #1-4 must be present for at least 6 weeks.

NODES AND NODULES IN RHEUMATIC DISEASE
1. Heberden's nodes→DIP osteophytes in 1° OA
2. Bouchard's nodes→ PIP osteophytes in 1° OA
3. Rheumatoid nodules
4. Gouty tophi (elbow, ears, heels, PIPs, DIPs)
5. Xanthomata

DDX OF MORNING STIFFNESS/PAIN WORSE IN AM
1. **Rheumatoid arthritis**
   - Difficulty doing up buttons
2. **Ankylosing Spondylitis**
   - LBP + stiffness radiating to buttocks and thighs
3. **PMR**
   - Difficulty getting out of bed
4. **Fibromyalgia**

CHARCOT'S JOINTS (NEUROPATHIC ARTHRITIDES)--ETIOLOGIES
1. Tabes dorsalis (spine; knees)
2. DM (feet)
3. Syringomyelia (shoulders, elbows); or
4. Overzealous intra-articular steroid injections

DDX OF ELBOW LESIONS
1. Rheumatoid nodule
2. Gouty tophus
3. Synovial cyst
4. Olecranon bursa (2° to gout, trauma)

5. Derm conditions…
    a) Psoriasis
    b) SQ calcification in CREST syndrome
    c) Tendon xanthoma

CLINICAL DIAGNOSIS OF SHOULDER PAIN

1. **Articular/Capsular disease**→All movements restricted
    a) 'Frozen shoulder' (aka adhesive capsulitis)
    b) Rheumatoid Arthritis
    c) Septic and other synovitis
2. **Rotator Cuff injury**
    a) Supraspinatus tendinitis
    b) Infraspinatus tendinitis (frequently see pain on active external rotation)
    c) Subscapularis tendinitis (frequently see pain on active internal rotation)
    d) Bicipital tendinitis (localized tenderness; frequently see pain on supination)

RADIOGRAPHIC SIGNS OF OSTEOARTHRITIS ✪

1. **Osteophyte** formation
2. **Subchondral sclerosis** (*no* periarticular osteopenia)
3. Joint space narrowing
4. Loose bodies
5. Sparing of MCP joints

RADIOGRAPHIC SIGNS OF RHEUMATOID ARTHRITIS ✪

1. **Periarticular osteopenia**
2. Symmetrical narrowing or the joint space
3. **Marginal bony erosions**
4. Subluxation and gross deformity

THERAPEUTIC EMERGENCIES IN RHEUMATIC DISEASE

1. **Atlanto-axial subluxation**
    Tends to affect RA patients on chronic steroids
    Treatment→Surgical decompression and fusion for progressive symptomatic disease
2. **Temporal Arteritis**
    Draw blood for ESR as soon as dx suspected
    Treat with high dose prednisone (60mg/day) as soon as ESR drawn
    Biopsy appearances are unaffected by ≤ 48hours of steroid therapy.
3. **Septic Arthritis**
    Drain joint; gram stain; C&S
    IV Abx
    Occasionally, arthroscopic debridement may be necessarily, e.g. if poorly responsive to Abx

4. Vasculitic Complications

   a. Mononeuritis Multiplex; digital gangrene; bowel infarction
   b. High-dose steroids; cytotoxic drugs; surgery

5. Iridocyclitis

   ♦ May complicate seronegative spondyloarthropathy (but *not* RA)

6. Episcleritis

   ♦ May complicate RA (but not seronegative spondyloarthropathies)

EXTRA-ARTICULAR MANIFESTATIONS OF R.A. : <u>"CLEAN SPUDS"</u>→
(more common in patients with <u>high titres</u> of RF)

C ardiac

L ymphadenopathy; ***Leukocytoclastic vasculitis*** (small vessel vasculitis)→palpable
   purpura; **L**ow pleural fluid glucose. Leukocytosis

E <u>p</u>iscleritis (usually treated topically)
A nemia (normocytic), Amyloidosis

N europathies (e.g. ***<u>Mononeuritis Multiplex</u>***)

S jogren's syndrome (***keratoconjunctivitis sicca***, or 2° Sjogren's, is the #1 opthalmic
   complication)

P ulmonary infiltration→fibrosis; <u>P</u>leurisy; obstructive lung dz of RA is associated with
   keratoconjunctivitis sicca; **P**neumoconiosis→large nodules (***Caplan's syndrome***);
   <u>P</u>ericarditis
U lcerated legs; <u>U</u>veitis

D igital vasculitis

S kin <u>nodules</u> (caused by endarteritis, a form of vasculitis)

- *Remember*: **Palpable Purpura almost always suggests an antecedent
   leukocytoclastic vasculitis.**

NOTES ON ASA and NSAIDs→common PRECAUTIONS/INTERACTIONS on boards:

- ASA→ Decreases metabolism of **oral hypoglycemics and therefore ↓s glu values!**

- Most **NSAIDs**→diminish the effects of **anti-HTN meds**

- While ASA *irreversibly* inhibits cyclooxygenase, NSAIDs *reversibly* inhibit the enzyme.

DMARD Therapy for RA		
DMARD	**Potential Toxicities Requiring F/U**	**Monitoring Studies**
Azathioprine	Myelosuppression, hepatotoxicity, lymphoproliferative disorders	CBC
Chlorambucil	Myelosuppression, myeloproliferative disorders, malignancy	CBC
Corticosteroids (PO prednisone, others.)	HTN, ↑glucose, osteoporosis	Baseline BP, chem pael, lipid profile, bone densitometry in high-risk patients; f/u glucose and lipids as indicated
Cyclophosphamide	Myelosuppression, myeloproliferative disorders, malignancy, hemorrhagic cystitis	CBC, urinalysis, and urine cytology
Cyclosporine	Renal insufficiency, anemia, HTN, hirsutism	Creatinine, CBC, K+, LFTs
Penicillamine	Myelosuppression, proteinuria	CBC and urine dipstick for protein
Etanercept (Enbrel®) (a TNF α-blocker)	Reactions at site of SQ injection, flu-like sx	none
Gold IM and PO	Myelosuppression, proteinuria	CBC and urine dipstick for protein
Hydroxycholorquine	Macular damage	Yearly opthalmologic exams
Infliximab (Remicade®)	Flu-like sx, auto-Abs; for patients not responding to methotrexate; given IV	none
Leflunomide (Arava®)	Thrombocytopenia, hepatotoxicity, diarrhea	CBC and AST
Methotrexate	Myelosuppression, hepatic fibrosis, cirrhosis, pulmonary infiltrates or fibrosis	CBC, AST, albumin
Minocycline	Photosensitivity, skin discoloration, GI upset, drug-induced hepatitis, dizziness	none
Sulfasalazine	Myelosuppression	CBC, AST, creatinine

✪ **Some of the More Commonly Used DMARDs Can be Remembered Using ⇒ "GOLD SCAM":**

Gold   (Most common toxicity is diarrhea)

S →   **ulfasalazine**

C →   **yclophosphamide** (e.g. treatment of **Wegener's**; works by ↓ing B cells, T cells; beware that its metabolite, acrolein, is toxic and can lead to hemorrhagic cystitis, which can be prevented with the use of MESNA; other toxicities include infertility, teratogenicity, and bone marrow suppression); **C**yclosporine; **C**orticosteroids.

A →   **ntimalarial** drugs (e.g. **hydroxycholorquine→retinopathy** is the major toxicity; clinical response to hydroxycholorquine may not be seen for 2-6 months after initiating); also **A**zathioprine (↓ dose by half if used in simultaneously with *allopurinol*)

M →   **ethotrexate** (good combination of efficacy and tolerability as seen in **RA**; however, GI toxicity #1 side effect; **CBC, LFTs, PFTs** all should be monitored; beware that **cryptic cirrhosis** may develop **without** ↑LFTs; interstitial lung disease and fibrosis may lead to **↓DLCO on PFTs; however, this can also be 2° to RA itself!**)

DMARDs (Disease-modifying antirheumatoid drugs): 2 KEY POINTS:

1. Do not wait to start patients on DMARDs until after they have failed multiple courses of NSAIDs. Begin therapy with DMARDs as soon as the diagnosis of RA is confirmed.
2. Methotrexate is the DMARD of choice in patients with severe disease. Start therapy with 7.5 mg weekly and raise the dosage at 1- or 2-month intervals until peak efficacy is achieved.

RA VS. OA—QUICK DIFFERENTIATORS

1. RA→predominant DIP involvement rare
   OA→ predominant MCP involvement rare

2. RA→disease manifestations include ulnar deviation at the MCPs OA→ disease manifestations include 1st carpometacarpal joint involvement (clinically and radiographically), and larger, weight-bearing joints (e.g. hips, knees, shoulders)

STILL'S DISEASE

1. Systemic onset juvenile R.A.
2. High spiking fevers; arthralgias/arthritis; seronegativity (-RF; -ANA); ↑WBC; macular rash; serositis; LN; H/SM

> ✪ **Triad** of Still's however, is the **F**ever, the **A**rthritis, and the **R**ash (*FAR*): Think "Board scores are *STILL FAR* away"

DIAGNOSIS OF <u>FELTY'S</u> SYNDROME

1. *Triad of ✪…*
   a) **Neutropenia**
   b) **Seropositive RA, plus**
   c) **Splenomegaly, plus**

2. Frequent concomitants
   a) Serious infections
   b) Leg ulcers
   c) Mononeuritis Multiplex
   d) Anemia, thrombocytopenia
   e) LN, Hepatomegaly
   f) Sjogren's syndrome
   g) Weight loss

3. Laboratory clues
   a) ↓WBC and ↓ platelets (2° to splenic sequestration)
   b) ↓ serum Complement
   c) + ANA, high titre RF (IgM)

4. Response to splenectomy (Recurrent life-threatening infection or life-threatening hemolytic anemia are indications for splenectomy)
   a) Arthritis not affected
   b) ↓WBC frequently improves, though only temporarily

✪ STILL'S VS. FELTY'S: A SELECTIVE COMPARISON:

STILL'S DISEASE	FELTY'S SYNDROME
↑WBC	↓WBC
Fever	No fever necessary
Seronegative RA	Seropositive RA
Splenomegaly	Splenomegaly

✪ DDX OF ORAL + GENITAL ULCERATION
1. Behcet's syndrome → Painful
2. E. multiforme → Painful
3. HSV → Painful
4. Pemphigus → Painful
5. Crohn's disease → Pain*less*
6. Reiter's syndrome → Pain*less*
7. Syphilis → Pain*less*

DIFFERENTIATING REITER'S VS. BEHCET'S

Feature	Reiter's	Behcet's
M:F	10:1	2:1
Ulcers	Painless	Painful
Predominant ocular disease	Conjunctivitis	Uveitis
Long-term ocular disability	rare	also rare
Long-term joint disability	frequent (50%)	rare
Spondylitis/sacroiliitis	frequent	rare
HLA association	B27	B12, B5 (esp ocular disease and colitis)
Important in pathogenesis	Infection is	Racial factors are
Treatment	NSAIDs	Immunosuppressives

CLINICAL SPECTRUM OF BEHCET'S SYNDROME
1. Ocular disease—occurs in 80%; more common in HLA B5 and Japanese men
2. Genital ulcers
3. E. nodosum (F>M; assoc'd with non-deforming arthritis); occur in 80%
4. Oral ulcers (98%)
5. Thrombophlebitis (30%)
6. CNS disease (30%)
   a) Aseptic meningitis
   b) TIA-like episodes
   c) Cranial nerve palsies
7. Colitis (30%)
   a) Assoc'd with HLA-B5
   b) May lead to perforation
   c) Clinically overlaps with IBD
8. Spondylits, sacroiliitis
   - When present, linked to IILA-B27

DIAGNOSTIC CRITERIA FOR PMR (Polymyalgia Rheumatica)
1. Age > 50
2. ESR > 40 mm/h
3. Neck/bilateral shoulder/pelvic girdle AM **stiffness**
   a) Symptomatic episodes >1h in duration
   b) Clinical history >1 month duration
4. Response to low-dose (≤15 mg/day) steroids
5. Minor criteria include:
   a) Weight loss; fever; night sweats
   b) Symmetrical proximal muscle tenderness
   c) ↑alk phos/GGT
   d) Normocytic anemia
   e) Synovitis
   f) Normal CPK, EMG, muscle biopsy

EXCLUSION OF COEXISTING TEMPORAL ARTERITIS (Giant Cell Arteritis)

1. **Presentation (classical) of Temporal Arteritis**→ H/A; **scalp tenderness; jaw claudication**; sudden visual loss.
2. **50%** of TA patients have symptoms of PMR
3. **10-20%** of patients with *clinically pure* PMR (i.e. only symptoms of PMR) will be found to have TA on biopsy.
4. 50% of *all* PMR patients (± TA symptoms) will be found to have giant-cell arteritis on TA biopsy.

> ⊗ **Remember, PMR patients complain more of *stiffness* than pain.**

5. False-negative biopsies may occur 2° to presence of '**skip lesions**' (if a 2cm biopsy is taken the false-neg rate is < 5%; therefore a **3-5cm segment biopsy** is recommended)
6. Height of initial ESR cannot be used to predict disease severity or likelihood of complications.

⊗ **IMPORTANT SIDE EFFECTS OF CHRONIC USE OF STEROIDS—for the exam...**
1. **Proximal myopathy**
2. **Avascular Necrosis (e.g. hip)**
3. **2° Osteoporosis**
4. Cataracts
5. Glucose Intolerance
6. Poor sleep; psychiatric changes
7. Striae
8. Weight gain

RELAPSING POLYCHONDRITIS

1. Associated with autoimmune disease in 30%
2. Leads to **fever, arthralgias, episcleritis, swollen floppy ears**
3. Nasal septum collapse (**the other 'saddle nose'** deformity, i.e. not just Wegener's)
4. **Laryngeal disease→hoarseness; respiratory obstruction** ⊗
5. Tracheobroncial degeneration→recurrent infections, respiratory arrest
6. AI/ MVP/Aneurysm in ~ 10%

RHEUMATOLOGIC MANIFESTATIONS OF SICKLE CELL DISEASE

1. Gout
2. Sickle crisis→lower extremity arthralgias, myalgias; synovitis
3. 2° hemochromatotic arthropathy (Fe overload 2° to frequent transfusions)
4. **Septic arthritis (or osteomyelitis), esp due to Salmonella**, particularly if hyposplenic.
5. Aseptic (avascular) necrosis.

GOUT

1. **Precipitating factors** common to gout and pseudogout include trauma, operation, alcohol

2. <u>**Conditions associated**</u> with gout: <u>**"HARD"**</u>→

   H TN
   A therosclerosis
   R enal stones
   D M

3. ✪ The hyperuricemia is either 2° to **OVERPRODUCTION** (→give <u>Allopurinol</u> or colchicine for prophylaxis) **or UNDEREXCRETION** (→give <u>Probenicid</u> for prophylaxis) or both. The way to distinguish the two is by ordering a <u>**24hour urine for uric acid levels**</u>. If high, then you have an overproducer. If low, patient is an underexcretor.

4. ✪ **NOTES ON TREATMENT:**

   a) **Colchicine** may give severe GI side effects in its PO form only

   b) **Indomethacin** (or other NSAID) should be *avoided in CHF and PUD*

   c) **Probenicid** is a uricosuric (↑s urinary secretion of uric acid) and should not be used if patient either has a h/o kidney stones or has a 24h U.A. level> 1000mg. Simultaneous administration of ASA or Indomethacin should be avoided if possible, as probenicid delays their excretion.

   d) <u>**Allopurinol should not be given for acute attacks**</u>. Instead give either colchicine or indomethacin

   e) <u>**Allopurinol is the drug of choice if patient has a h/o renal insufficiency or renal stones**</u>.

   f) Corticosteroids also very useful in mgmt.

   g) <u>**Allopurinol toxicities**</u>: "**FRREE**" (Fever, Rash, Renal, ↑eos, Elevated LFTs) as in "<u>FRREE</u> <u>Gout</u>" (but don't Freakout on the test!)…

      Fever
      Rash—Erythematous, desquamating
      Renal insufficiency
      Eos ↑
      Elevated LFTs

5. Uric acid crystals are <u>negatively birifringent</u>, as opposed to **P**seudogout, which is **P**ositively birifringent under polarized light microscopy. Remember 5-10% of patients will have both gout and pseudogout.

6. **For the exam, serum hyperuricemia is neither necessary nor sufficient to make the diagnosis of gout**. A synovial fluid aspirate is necessary for definitive diagnosis. Always remember, for definitive diagnosis, to send the synovial fluid for crystal analysis, gram stain, C&S. Nevertheless, the aspirations will not always reveal crystals either, so the absence of crystals does not necessarily rule out gout.

7. **Alcohol/diet/diuretics** are the most common cause of acute gout in the outpatient population.

8. Gout is very uncommon among premenopausal women.

CALCIUM PYROPHOSPATE DISEASE (CPPD)
1. **Associated diseases include**: hyperparathyroidism, hemochromatosis-hemosiderosis, hypothyroidism, gout, ↓Mg, ↓ Phos, and Wilson's disease.
2. When CPPD precipitates an acute inflammatory arthritis→it's called **"Pseudogout"**
3. Treatment options are similar to gout, except for allopurinol, of course.

HYDROXYAPATITE DEPOSITION DISEASE
1. Crystals are seen under transmission electron microscopy, and *not* polarized microscopy.
2. Can present either as an acute or chronic arthritis

SPONDYLOARTHROPATHIES

A. **DDx of Spondylitis**
   1. Ank Spond
   2. Other seronegative arthritides→psoriatic, Reiter's, juveline RA
   3. IBD; 'reactive' spondyloarthritis
   4. Infection
      a) Septic arthritis
      b) TB
      c) Brucellosis
B. **Characteristics ✪**:
   1. SI joint involvement
   2. Peripheral arthritis (usu asymmetric and oligarticular)
   3. Seronegativity (absence of RF)
   4. Association with HLA-B27
   5. Enthesopathy

C. **HLA-B27 Rheumatic Diseases ✪**:
   1. Ankylosing Spondylitits (>90% are HLA-B27+)
   2. Reiter's Syndrome or reactive arthritis (>80%)
   3. Enteropathic Spondylitis (75%)
   4. Psoriatic Spondylitis (50%)

D. An **offspring of a person with HLA-B27** has a 50% chance of inheriting the antigen.
E. Among **HLA-B27 persons in the general population**, only 2-10% will develop disease.

F. **ANKYLOSING SPONDYLITIS**

   1. **LBP**
      a) Onset between 15-40yo
      b) Insidious
      c) <u>**Early AM back stiffness**</u>
      d) Improves with exercise

   2. **Radiographic findings**
      a) Erosions
      b) Syndesmophytes
      c) <u>**'Bamboo spine'**</u>

   3. <u>**Enthesopathic**</u> **involvement**
      a) Plantar fasciitis
      b) Achilles tendinitis
      c) Costochondritis

   4. <u>**Iritis**</u> (an important clue in spondyloarthropathies)

   5. **Among the differentials of ank. spond. is** <u>**DISH**</u> ✪ ('Diffuse Idiopathic Skeletal Hyperostosis', *a form of 1° osteoarthritis*)

      a) Patients with DISH are often obese and 60% have diabetes;
      b) **Sensation of 'stiffness' at the spine, yet relatively well-preserved spinal motion;**

      c) **Criteria for DISH...**

          (1) <u>**'Flowing' ossification along the anterolateral aspects of ≥4 contiguous vertebral bodies with preservation of disk height**</u>
          (2) No apophyseal joint involvement
          (3) Absence of SI joint involvement
          (4) Extraspinal ossification

      d) <u>**Marked calcification and ossification of paraspinous ligaments**</u> occur in DISH. <u>**Ligamentous calcification and ossification in the anterior spinal ligaments give the appearance of "flowing wax"**</u> on the anterior vertebral bodies. However, **a radiolucency may be seen between the newly deposited bone and the vertebral body, differentiating DISH from the marginal osteophytes in spondylosis.**

      e) Intervertebral disk spaces are preserved, and sacroiliac and apophyseal joints appear normal, **helping to differentiate DISH from spondylosis and from ankylosing spondylitis**, respectively.

      f) The radiographic changes are generally much more severe than might be predicted from the mild symptoms.

6. **Spinal fracture is the #1 cause of death and disability** in Ank Spond 2°
to relatively minor trauma to a rigid spine.

7. *Don't be fooled*→ **HLA-B27 is *neither necessary not sufficient* for the dx**.

G. REITER'S SYNDROME ✪

1. Spondyloarthropathy PLUS
2. **Urethritis/Conjunctivitis** ±
3. Dysentery ±
4. **Circinate Balanitis** (rash on glans penis)/oral ulcers/keratoderma
5. **Keratoderma Blenorrhagicum** (indistinguishable clinically and histologically from psoriasis)
6. **Dactylitis ('sausage-like' digits)→can also be seen in Psoriatic Arthritis**

H. REACTIVE ARTHRITIS

1. An aseptic arthritis induced by host response to infectious agent rather than direct infection.

2. Follows **infections of GI and GU systems**. The organisms that trigger it are:
   a) Salmonella, Shigella flexneri
   b) Yersinia enterocolytica
   c) Campylobacter jejuni
   d) Ureaplasma Urealyticum

3. Clinical features of Reiter's may ensue.

I. ARTHRITIS ASSOCIATED WITH IBD

1. A non-deforming asymmetric arthritis, principally affecting knees, ankles, and PIPs, occurs in approximately 15%.

2. This **PERIPHERAL** arthitis tends to occur ≥ 6 months after the onset of bowel disease. Its **severity reflects/parallels that of the bowel disease** ✪. Colectomy rids it.

3. E. nodosum, uveitis, oral ulcers and pyoderma **occur in association with peripheral arthritis** in IBD.

4. **Spondylitis/Sacroiliitis** (considered more **CENTRAL** arthritis) occur in ~ 5%, may predate the onset of bowel symptoms, and are **associated with HLA-B27**. They are **independent of bowel disease activity** ✪, and so unaffected by colectomy.

5. Among patients with IBD + Ank Spond, ~75% are HLA-B27 +.

6. However, patients with IBD alone do not have an ↑d frequency of HLA-B27, nor do they have higher risk for developing spondylitis.

J. **PSORIATIC ARTHRITIS**
- *Of patients with psoriasis, only 7% develop the arthritis.*

CLINICAL PATTERNS:

1. *Oligoarticular, asymmetric type* (70%)→see **'sausage digits' (dactylitis),** which represents flexor tendon sheath effusions (**dactylitis also seen in Reiter's**)

2. *DIP joint type* (15%)→usually seen in assn with psoriatic **nail disease** (i.e. pitting and onycholysis); **pitting of the nails is strongly associated with joint disease**

3. *Pseudorheumatoid type*
   a) Seronegative
   b) M=F
   c) Severity of arthritis correlates with severity of **skin disease**

4. *Ankylosing Spondylitis type*
   - **HLA-B27 positive in >90%** only (less common than in 1° Ank Spond or Reiter's)

5. *Arthritis Mutilans*
   a) **Sacroiliitis** often assoc'd
   b) **'Telescoping digits'** (radiographically 'pencil-in-cup' appearance)

LYME DISEASE

1. Caused by the spirochete bacteria ***Borrelia Burgdorferi***, which is carried by the ***Ixodes dammini*** tick (the vector)
2. It is seen primarily in **summer and fall**

---

3. ✪ **Very early Lyme disease (4-6 weeks post-exposure) may show negative serology, so the patient's history, flu-like symptomatology, and ECM rash become critical in deciding whether or not to treat.**

---

4. *Stages:*
   Stage I
   a) 3-32 days after the tick bite
   b) Flu-like illness
   c) **ECM (Erythema Chronicum Migrans; 60%)**

   Stage II
   a) Weeks to months following bite
   b) 10-15% develop neurologic abnormalities (e.g. **Bell's palsy**) and/or carditis;
   c) **Arthritis develops in 30-50%**

Stage III

- **Arthritis develops in 50%**
    a) Can become chronic;
    b) Synovium resembles that of rheumatoid arthritis;
    c) Unique feature of lyme arthritis is **obliterative endarteritis** of synovium
    d) Those with chronic joint disease have ↑ frequency of **HLA-DR4**

5. Carditis and facial palsy are commonly reversible; prognosis is usually favorable

6. ✪ **Lyme test should be used only for confirmation if suspect the disease, and not for screening**, because of false positives and false negatives. False positives may be seen with infectious **mono, RA, SLE, and other spirochetal** disease. If suspect a false positive and/or the patient has one of these diagnoses→√ Western blot

7. *Complications by system…*

    a) Skin lesions (ECM)
    b) Neurological –Cranial nerve palsies; peripheral neuropathies; meningitis
    c) Cardiac—AV block; myopericarditis
    d) *Arthritis—recurrent, asymmetric; often affects the knee.*

8. *Treatment:*

    a) Early (ECM)→Doxy or Amox or Biaxin X 2-3 wk; or Cefuroxime x3 wk
    b) Carditis→Ceftriaxone/Cefotaxime/PenG X 2-3 weeks IV
    c) Facial nerve paralysis→Doxy or Amox X 3-4 weeks
    d) Meningitis→Ceftriaxone IV x 3weeks
    e) Arthritis→Doxy or Amox—duration unknown
    f) Pregnant women→No doxycycline!

✪ HYPERTROPHIC PULMONARY OSTEOARTHROPATHY (HOA)

1. Presentation also similar to RA

2. **Periosteal new bone formation** occurs at the end of long bones, giving **tenderness and soft-tissue swelling.**

3. This renders a so-called **spongy sensation** on palpation of the fingernail beds.

4. If lower extremities involved, **lowering the legs characteristically improves the pain.**

5. Usually 2° to **lung carcinoma or bacterial endocarditis**

CAUSES OF <u>C</u>LUBBING: " 7 C'S "→

C ardiac: SBE; cyanotic congential heart disease

C hest: cystic fibrosis; empyema; bronchiectasis; lung ca; TB (if extesive fibrosis); abscess

C rohn's disease; celiac disease; cirrhosis

C irculatory: AV fistula in upper extremities

C arcinoma: gastric, etc.

C ongenital clubbing

C ervical rib (unilateral)

Plus : thyrotoxicosis

AVASCULAR NECROSIS OF BONE
1. Associated conditions include
   a) Alcohol
   b) **chronic steroid use** ✪
   c) SLE and other connective tissue diseases
   d) Hemoglobinopathies, e.g. Sickle Cell disease
2. **Hip involvement** (at least on the exam)
3. **MRI** is best diagnostic tool on the exam! ✪

INFLAMMATORY MYOPATHIES
- Muscle biopsy is mandatory in each of these.
- **Polymyositis and Dermatomyositis→proximal muscle weakness** (e.g. rising from chair, brushing hair, or walking up the stairs); similar to steroids in this respect.
- Speaking of which, steroids are the treatment of PM and DM, until the CPK normalizes.
- Dermatomyositis→**heliotrope rash; Gottren's papules**
- **Inclusion Body Myositis**; unique in these respects ✪…
   a) Responds poorly to steroids
   b) Proximal *and distal* muscle involvement

COMPLEMENT LEVELS IN RENAL VS. SYSTEMIC DISEASE

	↓ **Serum C′**	**Normal Serum C′**
Primary renal dz	Poststrep GN MPGN (membrano- proliferative)	Berger's Dz (IgA) Alport's Syndrome **R**PGN (p- or c-ANCA+) "BAR"
Systemic disease	**S**LE **I**nfective Endocard **M**ixed essential cryo "SLIM *down*"	**G**oodpasture's Dz **H**US/TTP **O**ccult Abscess **S**ystemic Vasculitis (Wegener's; PAN; HSP) "GHOST"

SYSTEMIC LUPUS ERYTHEMATOSIS (SLE) ✪

A. **SLE Renal Disease**
 1. Mesangial changes alone→No aggressive treatment needed
 2. Active diffuse, proliferative GN→High-dose steroids ± immunosuppressives
 3. Focal proliferative GN and membranous GN→treatment controversial/prognosis favorable; renal biopsy often helpful in directing therapy

> - So, **Proliferation/inflammation/necrosis/crescent** formation→all requireTx

B. **↓Total C' correlates with active disease.**
C. **↓CH50 complement levels in SLE→usually mean renal or skin disease.**
D. Anti ds DNA levels also fluctuate with disease activity in general.
E. SLE patients may show a **false-positive VDRL 2° to cross-reaction of an anti-phospholipid Ab to VDRL**.
F. Most (80%) of SLE patients with a false + VDRL have circulating **lupus 'anti-coagulant' (really a 'pro-coagulant', since predisposes to thrombotic disease)**

ANTI-NUCLEAR ANTIBODY FLUORESCENT PATTERNS ✪ :

Fluorescent Pattern	Antigen	Rheumatic Disease
Homogeneous/diuse	DNP*	SLE (chronic)
Rim, peripheral	DNA	SLE (acute)
Nucleolar	RNA	Scleroderma
Speckled	ENA**	MCTD, SLE, Polymyositis

* DNP=Deoxyribonucleoprotein
** ENA=Entractable nuclear antigens

RHEUMATOLOGIC AUTOANTIBODIES ✪:

- **Anti-dsDNA→SLE** (70% sensitivity; highly specific); **Anti-ssDNA**→SLE (100% sensitivity, low specificity)

- **Anti-Sm (Smith)**→SLE (30% sensitivity but highly specific *if* you see it)

- **Anti-RNP** (Ribonuclear protein)→**MCTD** (Mixed Connective Tissue Disease)

- Anti-<u>S</u><u>S</u>-A ('anti-Ro') and -B ('anti-La')→<u>S</u>jogren's <u>S</u>yndrome (also SLE)

- **Antihistone→Drug-induced SLE (hydralazine and procainamide)**

- Anti-<u>Scl</u>-70→<u>Scl</u>eroderma (diffuse)
- Anti<u>C</u>entromere→<u>C</u>REST

> ✪ Remember, **numerous drugs can cause a + ANA without ever resulting in the clinical syndrome of drug-induced lupus**. Hydralazine and procainamide are important and common exceptions. If a patient is clinically stable on one, say, procainamide for an arrythmia, and his ANA is 1:640, you need not discontinue the medicine based on the ANA alone, unless symptomatic for drug-induced lupus (fever, arthralgias, pleurisy).

> ✪ **Anti-Jo** (Ab vs histidyl-tRNA synthetase)→**Polymyositis; Dermatomyositis; and PM- and DM-related Interstitial Pulmonary Fibrosis.** Anti-Jo antibody is associated with PM and DM only 25% of the time. **Remember too, ~ 10% of patients >40 with PM and 30% with DM have an associated malignancy.**

CREST Syndrome:

C alcinosis cutis

R aynaud's phenomenon

E sophageal dysmotility

S clerodactyly

T elangietasias

SCLERODERMA (Systemic Sclerosis)

S tiffness and aching. Skin feels thick and inelastic

C alcinosis, sclerodactyly and telangiectasia (CREST variant)

L oss of weight

E levated pulmonary pressure (**pulmonary HTN 2° to interstitial pulmonary fibrosis → cor pulmonale.**) A significant $\downarrow$ **DLCO** can be present on PFTs despite normal CXR.

R aynaud's syndrome

O esophagus (dysphagia)

D yspnea (50%)

E SR $\uparrow$

R ecurrent ulcers: **R**aynaud's; **R**enal HTN (**TREAT SCLERODERMA HTN WITH AN ACE I**)

M outh: skin contracts. Muscle weakness

A rthritis, acrosclerosis

S jogren's syndrome

ANTIPHOSPHOLIPID ANTIBODY SYNDROME

> ◆ **Remember, Antiphospholipid antibodies include either lupus anticoagulant and anti-cardiolipin Ab. Therefore either of these could lead to Antiphospholipid Ab Syndrome.**

Common Clinical Manifestations ✪
1. <u>**Recurrent fetal loss**</u>
2. <u>**Thrombocytopenia**</u>
3. <u>**DVT**</u>
4. <u>**Arterial Thrombosis**</u>
    a) CVA; recurrent TIAs
    b) Extremity gangrene
    c) Visceral infarction
5. <u>**Livedo Reticularis**</u> (*not* 'Le Vida Loca')

Coagulation Labs:
1. PT is normal or ↑
2. PTT is ↑
3. ↑ Bleeding time

> 4. ✪ <u>**↑PTT is not corrected by adding normal plasma, i.e. 1:1 dilution test,**</u> (since antiphospholipid Ab is an inhibitor, not a factor deficiency, and won't be corrected by adding a control patient's clotting factors).

> 5. ✪ Remember lupus '*ANTI*-coagulant' (which is an antiphospholipid Ab of either IgG or IgM classes) <u>is actually a '*PRO*-coagulant', as clearly seen in this syndrome since it predisposes to DVT and arterial thrombosis</u> (IgG association> IgM association)

> 6. Since these 2 factor inhibitors are so closely related, anticardiolipin Abs (like the lupus anticoagulant) <u>cross react</u> with several negatively-charged phospholipids, accounting for many of the clinical findings.

RAYNAUD'S PHENOMENON
1. Abnormality in microvasculature
2. F>M
3. Usually not associated with connective tissue disease, unless ANA+
4. Definitive dx by skin capillary microscopy→shows torturous, dilated capillary loops
5. Treatment:
    a) Wearing gloves
    b) Biofeedback
    c) Nitrates
    d) Calcium Channel Blockers
    e) D/C smoking (similar to Buerger's Disease—see later)
    f) Beta-blockers are contraindicated, as will ↑ the spasm

6. **Differentiating 1° vs. 2° Raynaud's phenomenon…**

1° RAYNAUD'S	2° RAYNAUD'S
Females	Males and Females
All digits	**Single digit**, usually
Frequent attacks	Infrequent attacks
Can be precipitated by emotional stress	Not precipitated by emotional stress
Digital ulceration rare	**Common**
Livedo Reticularis common	Uncommon

Antiestrogenic and Estrogenic Activities of Raloxifene and Tamoxifen:		
Tissue	**Raloxifene**	**Tamoxifen**
Bone	E	E
Breast	AE	AE
CNS	AE	AE
Endometrium	AE	E
Liver	E	E
Vagina	AE	AE

Abbreviations:
    E=Estrogenic effect
    AE=Antiestrogenic effect

OSTEOPOROSIS
1. ↓ in bone mass usually in postmenopausal women 2° to ↓ estrogen levels
2. *Important 2° causes* ✪ that must be ruled out include…

    a) **Endocrine {↑steroids; ↑T4; ↑PTH 2° ↑ resorption; ↑ sugars (DM)}**
    b) Malignancy
    c) Immobilization
    d) **Prolonged use of Steroids or Heparin**
    e) **Alcoholism**; malabsorption
    f) Hypogonadism (↓LH and FSH)
    g) **Smoking; Alcohol; Obesity**

3. Calcium homeostasis is unaffected; *serum Ca is normal*.
4. *Bone densitometry* is the gold standard for diagnosis.
5. *Treatment*: Calcium; Vit D; Weight-bearing exercises; Estrogen asap after menopause—add Progesterone if uterus is intact; if contraindicated or high risk of complications, may **try Raloxifene (Evista®)→does not improve the hotflashes, but will lower the LDL**; ALSO cut out any tobacco/excess alcohol/extra weight.
6. Remember, an *obese white postmenopausal smoker has 4 risk factors* for developing osteoporosis.

BONE MINERAL DENSITY TESTING And The W.H.O. Diagnostic Criteria For Adult Women:	
CATEGORY	**CRITERIA**
Normal	BMD within 1 Standard Deviation of the young adult reference mean
Low bone mass (**osteopenia**)*	BMD **>1 SD** below the young adult mean
Osteoporosis*	BMD **≥2.5 SD** below the young adult mean
Severe (established) osteoporosis*	BMD **≥2.5 SD** below the young adult *mean in the presence of an osteoporotic fracture*.

* **Candidates for HRT/alendronate/calcitonin**

OSTEOMALACIA ✪

1. Considered in the differential of osteoporosis
2. *Failure of <u>M</u>ineralization* of the bone due to …
    a) ↓ Vit D
    b) Vit D resistance
    c) ↓ phosphate
    d) Abnormal bony matrix
3. *↓Ca, ↓Phos, ↑alk phos*
4. *<u>Pseudofractures</u>* (noted radiographically as "Looser's zones")
5. Obviously one can have both osteoporosis and osteomalacia.
6. AKA "rickets" in children
7. *<u>Renal osteodystrophy (2° hyperparathyroidism)</u>*
    a) Related to phosphate retention, ↓ vit D, and acidosis—all part of CRF
    b) Syndrome consists of…
        i) Osteitis fibrosa
        ii) Osteomalacia
        iii) Hyperparathyroidism
8. Similar to osteoporosis, Vit D and Calcium are important in treatment.

PAGET'S DISEASE ✪

1. *Bone is structurally weakened 2° to <u>disorganized bone remodeling</u>*
2. *<u>Normal serum Ca</u>* (similar to osteoporosis), except with immobilization
3. *↑alk phos (similar to osteomalacia) and it correlates with disease activity*.
4. Unknown cause
5. Affects axial>appendicular skeleton, with particular preference for:
    a) Sacrum
    b) Spine
    c) Femur
    d) Tibia
    e) Skull (lytic lesions here called osteoporosis circumscripta)
    f) Pelvis

6. Skeletal pain ;deformities; fractures
7. High Output cardiac failure
8. *↑Urinary hydroxyproline and ↑24 hour urine N-telopeptide are very useful markers*
9. Nuclear bone scans see "hot" spots of Paget's dz, and are far better than plain films in dx
10. *Potential for malignant transformation*, esp tumors of the humerus and femur)
11. Calcitonin and bisphosphonates (e.g. etidronate) commonly used in management.

Clinical Lab Data Associated with Common Metabolic Bone Diseases:

Bone Disorder	Serum calcium	Serum phosphorus	Alkaline phosphatase
Osteoporosis	N[1]	N	N
Osteomalacia	↓	↓	↑
Hyperparathyroidism	↑	↓	↑
Renal failure/ osteodystrophy	↓	↑	↑
Paget's Disease	N	N	↑↑

1. N = Normal

POPLITEAL CYST

1. *An extension of inflamed synovium into the popliteal space*; also known as a '**Baker's cyst**'

2. A **ruptured Baker's cyst** may resemble acute DVT, and has therefore also been referred to as '**pseudophlebitis**'

3. Ultrasound is typically the initial imaging modality of choice

4. **DDx** is primarily DVT; popliteal artery aneurysm; LNs; and tumor.

FIBROMYALGIA

♦ A diagnosis of exclusion

♦ F>>M

♦ Pain must be present for ≥ 3mo

♦ Multiple tender, painful points

♦ Patients are poorly able to localize their pain, which is ↑ in Ams

♦ Patients frequently do not feel rested on awakening

♦ Nervousness is a frequent concomitant.

VASCULITIDES ✪

PAN (Polyarteritis Nodosa)

A. *Common manifestations*
1. Abdominal pain/ischemic bowel→**abdominal aneurysms**

2. Focal necrotizing GN→**HTN**

3. **Palpable purpura and livedo reticularis**

4. **Mononeuritis multiplex** (similar to RA)

5. **Constitutional** sx's
   a) Fever
   b) Fatigue
   c) Weight loss
   d) Myalgia
   e) Arthralgia

6. ↑LFTs

> 7. **PAN**→ **p-AN**CA (as opposed to **We**gener's = **c-AN**CA—"**We cAN**"). However, in vasculitides, cannot rely on the ANCA for dx; need biopsy!

B. *Infrequent Manifestations*
1. Testicular pain
2. MI, CHF
3. CVA, Sz
4. Retinal hemorrhage
5. Interstitial pneumonitis

CRYOGLOBULINEMIA

A. **Type I**
1. Single, *monoclonal* antibody
2. Symptoms, if any, are usually related to **hyperviscosity**
   a. H/As
   b. Epistaxis
   c. Raynaud's phenomenon
   d. Ischemic ulcers
   e. Visual complaints
B. **Type II**
1. Commonly associated with **autoimmune disorders and chronic infections**
2. Usual presentation is **palpable purpura; urticaria; skin ulcers**; may also see arthralgias/arthritis and peripheral neuropathies
3. Over the long run, **progressive renal disease** is a common complication

CHURG-STRAUSS

1. **Asthma + peripheral eosinophilia**

2. *3 Stages* (need not occur in this order):

    a. Usually a prodrome of **upper respiratory** disease in the form of…

        i. Allergic rhinitis, or

        ii. Asthma

        iii. Nasal polyposis

    b. ↑ **Blood and tissue eos**

    c. Life-threatening **vasculitis**

BUERGER'S DISEASE

1. Seen in **young adult smokers**, M>F

2. Present with **instep claudication and digital infarction**

3. Pathology is intraluminal thrombus-containing microabscesses to small and mid-size arteries and veins

4. **Quitting smoking stops the disease** progression

WEGENER'S GRANULOMATOSIS

1. **Pulmonary-renal syndrome (others include** Goodpasture's; Churg-Strauss; SLE; Cryoglobulinemic vasculitis; Leukocytoclastic vasculitis, i.e. small vessel vasculitis)

2. Pulmonary manifestations include hemorrhage and thick-walled, centrally-**cavitating nodules**;

3. Renal manifestation is **Focal Segmental** GN

4. The mnemonic **ELKS** summarizes the organs affected:

    E NT

    L ung

    K idney

    S kin

5. <u>GASTROENTEROLOGY</u>

SOME LESIONS CAUSING CHRONIC, RECURRENT GI BLEEDING...

1. AVMs (arterial-venous malformations)
    a) remember, tend to affect <u>Right</u> side of colon and small bowel.
    b) ↑ incidence in <u>Aortic Stenosis</u>
    c) ↑ in dialysis and ESRD
    d) Treatment is usually cautery
2. Diverticulitis—including Meckel's.

HEMATEMESIS IN THE ALCOHOLIC...

1. Alcoholic gastritis
2. Mallory-Weiss syndrome
    a) mucosal laceration at EG junction
    b) 75% of patients have a history of retching and vomiting before bleeding.
4. Bleeding varices
5. PUD
6. Coagulopathy

RISK OF REBLEEDING IN PUD BASED ON HOW THE BLEED APPEARS AT ENDOSCOPY
1. *Clot visualized* overlying site of bleed→ 10-40% risk of rebleed→Observation
2. *No overlying clot* seen; *only flat spot* →0-10% risk of rebleed →Observation
3. *Culprit vessel visualized* on exam →50-70% risk of rebleed →Requires treatment via endoscopy (e.g. laser photocoagulation, sclerotherapy, etc)

COMMON CAUSES OF RECURRENT ALCOHOL-INDUCED ABDOMINAL PAIN...

1. Alcoholic hepatitis
2. Alcoholic gastritis/PUD
3. Alcoholic pancreatitis

RECURRENT ACUTE ABDOMEN OF UNCLEAR CAUSE...

1. Narcotic addiction (malingering)
2. Familial Mediterranean Fever
3. Acute intermittent porphyria
4. Sickle cell anemia
5. Lead poisoning
6. Medications

BLEEDING TENDENCY IN ALCOHOLIC CIRRHOSIS

1. *↓ Synthesis of coagulation factors (↑PT)*: remember, since the half life of factor VII is only 6hours, the PT is a sensitive index of hepatic function; albumin is the other important index of hepatic function. Sometimes, it is difficult to determine if a patient's ↑ PT is 2° to liver disease or ↓ vit K, so <u>remember</u> this trick: If factor 5 is ↓, it's liver disease; if Factor 5 is normal, vitamin K deficiency.

2. *Platelet function defect (↑bleeding time)*
   a) Cirrhosis-induced von Willebrand-type defect
   b) Separate alcohol-induced platelet function defect

3. *Thrombocytopenia*
   a) Hypersplenism
   b) Marrow suppression

4. *Local factors*
   a) Varices
   b) PUD
   c) Gastritis
   d) Mallory-Weiss tears

BOERHAAVE'S SYNDROME
1. Esophageal perforation which commonly occurs after *dilatation*
2. *Similar to Mallory-Weiss, it often follows violent retching*, as after an alcoholic binge.

HEPATOMEGALY + HEART FAILURE—not just CHF !
1. Alcoholic cardiomyopathy with fatty liver
2. Amyloidosis
3. Carcinoid syndrome
4. Constrictive pericarditis (Pulsus paradoxus, rapid "y" descent in JVD)
5. Hemochromatosis
6. Right ventricular failure ± tricuspid incompetence
7. Left heart failure (!) which is the #1 cause of right heart failure.

DDX OF FLAPPING TREMOR...
1. Hepatic encephalopathy
2. Wilson's Disease
3. Uremia
4. CO_2 narcosis

SUDDEN ↑ IN ASCITES IN PREVIOUSLY STABLE CIRRHOSIS
1. SBP (esp if fever/chills/abdominal pain)
2. Hepatic vein thrombosis (Budd-Chiari syndrome)

3. Hepatoma (hepatocellular carcinoma); √ alpha fetoprotein; re: Hep B and C carry ↑ risk of cirrhosis→hepatoma; Hep A does not.
4. Acute deterioration in hepatocellular function; e.g....
    a) Sepsis
    b) Hemorrhage
    c) Alcohol binge
5. Hepatorenal syndrome

IRRITABLE BOWEL SYNDROME (IBS)
1. ↑ # of bowel movements with ↑ **stress**;
2. Abdominal pain **relieved by defecation**. ***Pain in IBS does not awaken the patient from sleep.***
3. **Pencil-thin stools**
4. Chronic or recurrent abdominal **distension**; dyspepsia
5. Feeling of incomplete evacuation

GASTRINOMA
1. Fasting ↑ gastrin level
2. Paradoxical ↑ in serum gastrin following secretin infusion
3. UGI shows
    a) Ectopic ulceration
    b) Rugal hypertrophy; duodenal nodularity
    c) Hyperperistalsis
4. Tumor visualization with CT, U/S, or angiography

↑ ALK PHOS—FACTORS FAVORING HEPATIC ORIGIN
1. ↑GGT
2. ↑5'-nucleotidase
3. ↑ LDH-5 isoenzyme

MOST IMPORTANT LABORATORY INDICATORS OF LIVER FUNCTION:
1. Albumin
2. Prothrombin time

LABORATORY INDICATORS OF ALCOHOLIC LIVER DISEASE:
1. ↑GGTP
2. ↑MCV; macrocytosis
3. AST/ALT > 2:1 (remember, 'S' for Superior)
4. Blood alcohol (if suspect daily drinking)
5. AFP (if hepatoma suspected)

LABORATORY INVESTIGATION OF HEMOCHROMATOSIS

♦ *Serum* <u>TRANSFERRIN SATURATION</u>, *preferably in the fasting state, is the best initial <u>SCREENING</u>* test for hemochromatosis.

♦ In otherwise healthy persons, a fasting serum transferrin saturation **greater than 62 percent** suggests hemochromatosis.

♦ While iron-binding saturations of **>90% are typical**, hemochromatosis **should be suspected at levels about 50%, especially in women.**

♦ Serum ferritin > 1000

♦ ↑ serum Fe, reduced TIBC

♦ (also liver biopsy—grade 3 or 4 Fe stains)

GILBERT'S DISEASE

1. **#1 cause of isolated ↑ <u>Indirect</u> Bili, which is, in turn, the #1 cause of ↑ bili**
2. Usually caused by **fasting states** and resolves after patient has eaten.

UNDERSTANDING BILIRUBIN AND JAUNDICE

	Normal U.Urobilinogen	↑U. Urobilinogen
↑ Conjugated Bili (Direct)	Common Bile Duct Obstruction	Acute **H**epatitis
↑ UNconjugated Bili (Indirect)	**Gilbert's** Disease **Crig**ler-Najjar ("<u>**U**nder **G**ilbert's **cri**b</u>")	Hemolysis

HEPATITIS B SEROLOGY SIMPLIFIED ✪ …

1. + Hep BsAg (**surface antigen**)→ means <u>active infection</u>

2. + anti-HepBs (**surface antibody**) →means <u>recovery and immunity</u>

3. + Hep BeAg ('**e' antigen**) →means <u>patient is infectious</u>

4. + anti-HepBe means ('**e' antibody**) →usually means patient is <u>no longer infectious</u>

5. HepBcAg (**core antigen**) is not routinely detected in peripheral blood

6. + IgM anti-HBc (**core antibody**) →means <u>acute infection</u> with Hep B. It appears after Hep BsAg disappears.

7. Persistence of anti-HBc (**core antibody**) means <u>chronic infection</u>, especially chronic active hepatitis (CAH—not to be confuse with the other CAH, congenital adrenal hyperplasia!—see Endocrine lecture)

8. Hep BsAg (**surface antigen**) can be ordered first. If negative, order surface and core antibodies. <u>If the surface Ag or core Ab are + for more than 6 months</u> (serologically, chronic hepatitis—re: ↑ transaminases ≥ 6 mo is more commonly used to define "chronic hepatitis"), <u>request 'e' Ag and Ab to evaluate for infectivity.</u>

9. <u>If a chronic surface Ag carrier presents with unexplained exacerbation, request *delta agent antibody*. The delta agent is important in the conversion of chronic persistent →chronic active hepatitis, and is strongly associated with IV drug abuse.</u> Remember, CAH can be treated with alpha-interferon.

10. If see **<u>sudden ↑ in ascites</u>** in a patient with history of Hep B or C → **√ <u>alpha fetoprotein (hepatoma) and R/O SBP</u> (spontaneous bacterial peritonitis)**

11. If patient with **<u>chronic Hep B</u>** presents with **<u>new or sudden abdominal pain</u>** that cannot be accounted for by liver disease per se, R/O **PAN** (polyarteritis nodosa).

12. If a non-immune individual is exposed to Hep B, s/he may be protected by giving HBIG (**passive** Hep B immunoglobulin); but s/he will still require **active** immunization with a routine series of 3 shots can be given if patient is going to be continously exposed to the virus.

13. If patient not found to have Hep B (or **Hep C, which can simply be checked with Hep C antibody, although dx must be confirmed via a <u>RIBA</u>** for Hep C), then additional testing may be done for other causes of usually ↑ transaminases, including…
    a) Anti-smooth muscle antibody (ASmA)→Autoimmune Hepatitis
    b) Anti-mitochondrial antibody (AMA)→PBC
    c) ANA→non-specific
    d) ↓ Serum ceruloplasmin and ↑ 24h urinary Copper excretion →Wilson's dz
    e) Alpha-1-antitrypsin Ab→congenital emphysema

- ◆ **Natural history of HepC**: 50% of patients with HepC go onto become chronically infected, and 50% of *those* develop CAH; 20% develop cirrhosis; Re: Hep C is the #1 cause of post-transfusion hepatitis

- ◆ Remember to **R/O HepC in patients with isolated ↑ ALT.**

- ◆ **HepA** can go onto develop fulminant hepatitis (very rare), but never get chronic infection or cirrhosis.

✪ ASSOCIATIONS/COMPLICATIONS OF HEPATITIS **B** TO KNOW:

1. **Aplastic anemia**

2. *Glomerulonephritis*

3. *Hepatocellular carcinoma* (hepatoma)

4. *Polyarteritis nodosa (PAN)*

WHICH ONE WAS IT AGAIN, SG<u>O</u>T OR SG<u>P</u>T?
Remember, it's SG<u>O</u>T in the following…

- ◆ Remember, SGOT is also one of the <u>cardiac enzymes</u>
- ◆ <u>Ranson's criteria</u> uses AST (SGOT)
- ◆ <u>Tylenol toxicity</u> (SGOT >4000)

Perhaps you'll *remember*, **"<u>O</u>H, <u>NO</u>, not that again!"**

PHASES OF HEPATITIS B…

Active replicative phase **(acute hepatitis or chronic active hepatitis)**
1. + 'e' Ag; neg 'e' Ab→**CONTAGIOUS**
2. + HBV DNA

Intermediate phase
1. Replication ceases
2. Liver damage accelerates

Integrative phase
1. Neg 'e' Ag; + 'e' Ab→ **NON-CONTAGIOUS**
2. - HBV DNA
3. Surface Ag remains + usually, but not always
4. HBV DNA becomes integrated into the hepatocyte genome.

Goals of Antiviral Therapy in Chronic Hepatitis B

1. ↑ Survival
2. ↓ In symptoms
3. ↓ Infectivity
4. ↓ Risk of developing hepatocellular ca.
5. HBsAg→anti-HBs seroconversion
6. Interruption of progression to cirrhosis
7. Loss of serum and intrahepatic HBV DNA by PCR
8. Normalization of serum ALT
9. Resolution of hepatic inflammation
10. Sustained loss of HBV replication (HBeAg→anti-Hbe seroconversion/loss of HBV DNA)

DIAGNOSTIC TESTS FOR HEPATITIS C

Test	Purpose	Use	Comments
ELISA[1]	Detects anti-HCV Ab	Screening test	+ Results must be verified with supplemental assay
RIBA[2]	Detects anti-HCV Ab	Supplemental assay to confirm + screen	
Qualitative RT-PCR[3] amplification of HCV RNA	Detects circulating HCV RNA	1) Qualitative assay to confirm + screen 2) To monitor patients on antiviral therapy	Detects virus <1-2 wks after exposure Single negative result not conclusive

1. ELISA, enzyme-linked immunosorbent assay
2. RIBA, recombinant immunoblot assay
3. RT-PCR, reverse transcriptase polymerase chain reaction

✪ *Approach to HCV Testing*: It's best to start with ELISA for anti-HCV. If repeatedly reactive, check either a **RIBA or the RT-PCR**. If either is +, then the patient has HCV.

✪ Remember if the patient has a + ELISA and a + confirmatory RIBA for Hep C, but the PCR is negative, this indicates the patient had *PRIOR EXPOSURE* to Hep C infection.

HCV—WHICH TESTS TO ORDER AND WHEN !

Indication	**Test**
Screening	HCV Ab
Diagnosis	HCV Ab; Qualitative HCV RNA
Prognosis	None
Decision to treat	Qualitative HCV RNA
Treatment Schedule	HCV genotype; Quantitative HCV RNA
Response to Treatment	Qualitative HCV RNA

✪ DIAGNOSTIC TESTS FOR HEPATITIS C:

Category	**ALT**	**EIA**	**RIBA**	**HCV RNA** (RT-PCR)
False positive EIA	N	+	-	-
Resolved infection or	N	+	+	-
HCV Carrier	N	+	+	+
Chronic Hep C intermittent viremia	↑	+	+	+

✪ IMPORANT BASIC POINTS ON TESTING FOR HCV:

- First an EIA (Enzyme Immunosorbent Assay) antibody is done.

- **All positive EIA results must be confirmed with a supplemental assay such as the RIBA or qualitative RT-PCR.**

- In **low/no risk** patients, if EIA is +, √ for HCV RNA by PCR; if that's +, consider bx, tx, etc.

- If the patient is *at* **high/↑ risk** for HCV and the PCR is negative, a RIBA (RadioImmunoBlot Assay) should be done *to distinguish resolved infection vs. a false + EIA→* if the RIBA is +, this means the patient had the infection but has cleared the virus. If the RIBA is negative, the EIA was most likely a false +.

- Re also: Because some HCV-infected patients may be only intermittently HCV RNA +, a single negative test cannot be used to R/O chronic infection, and repeat testing at 3-6 mo intervals by PCR is indicated to check for *chronic infection with intermittent viremia*.

- Re: EIA and RIBA detect anti-HCV generally within 15 weeks of exposure, while qualitative RT-PCR detects presence of virus as early as 1-2 weeks post-exposure.

- **HCV GENOTYPE**: There are 6 genotypes. *Genotype 1 is the most common in the US and is associated with lower response rates to current therapy*.

CURRENT TREATMENT GUIDELINES IN HEP C	
(from the National Concensus Development Conference Panel Statement: management of Hep C)	
Patient Characteristics	**Recommendations**
Persistent HCV viremia; persistently ↑ ALT; & liver biopsy showing portal or bridging fibrosis or moderate inflammation or necrosis	Consider Rx with interferon and ribavirin
Persistently normal ALT	Observe
↑ ALT, minimal abnormalities in biopsy	Observe, serial ALTs, consider biopsy q3-5y
Compensated Cirrhosis	Observe, consider treatment
Decompensated cirrhosis	Consider liver transplant

COUNSELING PERSONS WITH POSITIVE HCV TEST RESULTS: *ADVISE PATIENTS...*

- ◆ Not to drink alcohol
- ◆ To be vaccinated vs. Hep A and B
- ◆ Not to donate blood, organs, tissue, semen
- ◆ Not to share dental appliances, razors, or other items that might contain blood
- ◆ To cover cuts, sores on the skin
- ◆ To discuss with long-term, steady sex partners the low but not absent risk of transmitting HCV infection; to mention to these partners that they can use latex condoms, if they wish, to ↓ this low risk even further, and to discuss the possibility of being tested for HCV
- ◆ To talk with their physician before taking any new meds, including OTCs and herbals.

DISEASE PROGRESSION IN CHRONIC HEP C:

Chronic Hepatitis ⟶ **Cirrhosis** ⟶ **Hepatocellular Ca** ⟶ **Death**

20-30years   5-10years   variable

- • Acute infection goes onto chronic infection >85% of the time
- • Chronic infection leads to cirrhosis in 20-40% of cases
- • Hep C patients with decompensated cirrhosis should not be treated with interferon but should be considered for liver transplantation.
- • Hepatitis A and B vaccines are recommended for all patients with Hep C

REMEMBER THE 'RULE OF 20s' WITH HEP C:

- ◆ *20%* of patients with acute Hep C have *symptoms*
- ◆ 15-*20%* of patients with acute Hep C *clear the virus*
- ◆ In *20%* to 40% of patients with chronic Hep C, *cirrhosis* develops over *20* years
- ◆ Cirrhosis leads to *liver failure* in *20%* of these patients, and to *HCC* in another *20%*
- ◆ *20%* of patients without cirrhosis who receive *interferon* will obtain a *sustained response*.

PREVENTING HEP C TRANSMISSION—GUIDELINES FROM THE NIH

1. Adherence to universal precautions to protect medical personnel and patients against HCV should be sufficient.
2. Advise patients with HCV infection not to donate blood, organs, tissues, or semen
3. Strongly encourage safer sexual practices, including the use of latex condoms, in patients with multiple sexual partners.
4. The risk of transmission is low (<3%) in monogamous long-term relationships; therefore, no changes in sexual practices are recommended to these individuals
5. HCV Ab testing is recommended for the sex partners of infected patients.
6. Advise patients not to share razors and toothbrushes. Covering an open wound is recommended. However, it is not recommended to avoid close contact with family members or to avoid sharing meals or utensils.
7. Pregnancy is not contraindicated in women with HCV infection. The risk of transmission to the fetus is low (3-6%)
8. There is no evidence of transmission during breastfeeding; thus, breast-feeding is considered safe and should be encouraged.

✪ EXTRAHEPATIC MANIFESTATIONS OF CHRONIC HCV INFECTION

1. *Porphyria cutanea tarda*
2. *Cryoglobulinemia, type II*
3. *Leukocytoclastic vasculitis*
4. *Membranoproliferative GN*
5. Thyroiditis
6. Sjogren's Syndrome
7. Lichen Planus
8. B-Cell Lymphoma; plasmacytoma

DISTINGUISHING <u>COINFECTION</u> VS. <u>SUPERINFECTION</u> WITH HDV

	Hepatitis B	**Hepatitis D**
Coinfection	Surface Ag + ore IgM+	Hep D Ab+
Superinfection	Surface Ag+ core IgM-	Hep D Ab+

NOTES:

- HDV is an RNA virus that is unable to replicate on its own and requires HBV

✪ **HDV can occur as a "*superinfection*" in patients with underlying *chronic* HBV or as a "coinfection" during acute HBV infection.**

✪ The major significance of HDV is its ability to ↑ the severity of HBV infection. For example, fulminant hepatitis is more likely in patients who have acute HBV with HDV coinfection. And patients with chronic HBV who become superinfected with HDV may have an acute worsening of liver disease and a more rapid progression to cirrhosis.

Typical Transaminase Ranges for Various Diseases:

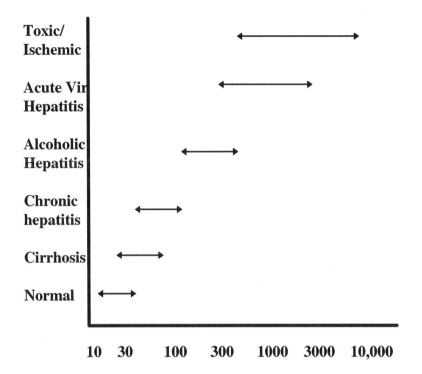

HEPATITIS E
1. Enterically transmitted
2. Resembles hep A
3. If a *woman in her 3rd trimester* acquires hep E→ high risk of going onto fulminant hepatitis.

AUTOIMMUNE HEPATITIS ✪
1. *Young women, primarily; average 10-20 yo*
2. ↑↑serum gamma globulins
3. + ANA
4. + <u>anti-Smooth muscle Ab;</u> *have been associated with* <u>anti-LKM</u> (liver-kidney-microsomal antibodies) and <u>soluble liver antigen.</u>
5. Treatment is *steroids*

ALCOHOLIC HEPATITIS ✪
1. A histological diagnosis (e.g. *Mallory bodies*, etc)
2. Clinical: N/V; anorexia; abdominal pain; ↓ weight
3. #1 sign is hepatomegaly
4. ↑AST (*AST/ALT >2/1*)
5. Poor prognosticators: spider nevi; ↑ PT; bili>20; renal failure; ascites; encephalopathy.

PRIMARY BILIARY CIRRHOSIS (PBC) ✪

1. Idiopathic disease of *middle-aged women*
2. Affects the small bile ducts
3. ↑*alk phos* and ↑ IgM; + *AMA (anti-mitchondrial antibody)*
4. *Pruritis*, steatorrhea (2° to progressive cholestasis)
5. Treatment: ursodeoxycholic acid (*UDCA*); colchicine.

PRIMARY SCLEROSING CHOLANGITIS ✪

1. Larger bile ducts (extra and intrahepatic) suffer an obliterative inflammatory **fibrosis**
2. Also felt to be autoimmune
3. Dx→Cholangiography
4. *Ulcerative Colitis associated* in 70% of cases (may come before, during, or after the PSC)
5. ↑*risk of cholangiocarcinoma* (bile duct ca)
6. Treatment is primarily supportive, although many patients require liver transplant.

ALCOHOL-INDUCED LIVER DISEASE→"*SMASH*" (as in: an alcoholic might get "smashed")

1. **S** teatohepatitis (fatty liver)—dose dependent; reversible
2. **M** icronodular cirrhosis
3. **A** lcoholic hepatitis (precursor for cirrhosis)
4. **S** iderosis, hepatic
5. **H** epatocellular carcinoma (hepatoma)

ORAL CONTRACEPTIVE USE AND LIVER DISEASE ✪

1. **Adenomas ± intraperitoneal rupture** (also seen in pregnancy)
2. **Cholelithiasis**
3. **Cholestasis**
4. **Focal nodular hyperplasia**
5. **Hepatic vein thrombosis**
6. **Peliosis Hepatis** (*blood-filled cysts in the liver*)

PELIOSIS HEPATIS, ASSOCIATIONS WITH...

1. **OCPs**

2. **Pregnancy**

3. **Anabolic steroids (also ↑ risk of angiosarcoma)**

4. **Bartonella henselae (re: cause of cat-scratch disease and bacillary angiomatosis)**

MORE USEFUL MNEMONICS..

IMPORTANT CAUSES OF CIRRHOSIS→ "*ABCDEF*":

A lpha-1-antitrypsin deficiency
B udd Chiari Syndrome, Hep B
C: Hep C
D rugs
E thanol
F e overload (iron overload)

LIVER DYSFUNCTION IN IBD→ "*CCCHHH*"

C holelithiasis in Crohn's disease (re: "stones in Crohn's)
C holangiocarcinoma
C holangitis (either pericholangitis—usually minimally symptomatic ↑alk phos—or *sclerosing cholangitis*)
H epatitis (CAH)→cirrhosis; granulomatous)
H epatic infiltration (fat, amyloid)
H epatic vein thrombosis

HEPATIC VEIN THROMBOSIS MAY COMPLICATE THESE ✪ →"*HOPPING*"

H epatoma
O CPs—as noted above
P NH
P Vcra
I BD-as noted above
N ephro**G**enic carcinoma (renal cell ca)

FATTY LIVER MAY BE CAUSED BY ✪ →"*PIC-A-DOT*"; *or remember you have to store all your excesses somewhere! …*

P regnancy (↑β-HCG)
I BD (↑ inflammation)
C ushing's syndrome (↑cortisol)
A lcohol (↑Etoh)
D M (↑ glucose)
O besity (↑ fat)
T hyrotoxicosis (↑thyroxine)

BASIC IMAGING MODALITIES IN SUSPECTED GALLBLADDER DISEASE

1. *Oral cholecystography→*
   - Used to demonstrate gallstones in anicteric patients when U/S is either unavailable or inconclusive
2. *U/S→*
   - Can distinguish obstructive from hepatocellular jaundice by demonstrating bile duct dilatation
3. *HIDA scan→*
   - High sensitivity and specificity for acute cholecystitis: cystic duct obstruction prevents gallbladder visualization.
4. *ERCP→*
   - Useful in postcholecystectomy jaundice
   - Helps to exclude false negatives from #1 or #2 above
   - Localizes obstruction within pancreatic or common bile duct (choledocholithiasis).
5. *PTC (Percutaneous transhepatic cholangiogram)→*
   - Localizes obstruction when intrahepatic ducts are dilated.

NONOPERATIVE THERAPIES FOR SYMPTOMATIC GALLSTONES:		
Agent	**Results**	**Notes**
Oral bile acid dissolution: (ursodeoxycholic acid=Actigall)	30-90 % successful dissolution; no mortality	50% recurrence rate; dissolves noncalcified cholesterol stones; *optimal for stones <5mm;*
Contact solvents: methyl *tert*-butyl ether/*n*-propyl acetate	50-90%	70% recurrence rate; duodenitis, hemolysis, nephrotoxicity, mild sedation
Lithotripsy	70-90%	70% recurrence rate; selection criteria→*no more than 1 radiolucent stone <20mm* in diameter, patent cystic duct, functioning gallbladder in a patient with symptomatic stones without complications

ACHALASIA IMAGING ✪ *(mechanism is the incomplete relaxation of the LES)*
1. **"Bird's beak" sign** on UGI (dilated esophagus with tapered lower end)
2. Tertiary contractions replacing peristaltic activity at all levels (manometry confirms a diagnosis made on UGI)
3. Absent gastric A/F (air/fluid) level
4. Intrathoracic A/F level

GIANT GASTRIC RUGAE
1. **Malignancy** (e.g. lymphoma, leiomyoma)
2. **Gastrinomas**

SYNDROMES OF MULTIPLE INTESTINAL POLYPS Commonly Addressed On The Exam...
1. Familial polyposis
2. Gardner's syndrome
3. Peutz-Jeghers syndrome

DIAGNOSIS OF LACTOSE INTOLERANCE
1. History of loose bm's/flatulence/cramps after milk products
2. Successful therapeutic trial of milk-free diet
3. Positive hydrogen breath test following oral lactose.

IMPORTANT INDICATIONS FOR SMALL BOWEL BIOPSY
1. Celiac Disease
2. Whipple's disease (re: infiltration or replacement of lamina propria with foamy *PAS-positive macrophages*)
3. Nodular lymphoid hyperplasia
4. Crohn's disease
5. Lymphoma
6. Parasites
   a) Giardia
   b) Strongyloides
7. Fungi
   a) Candida
   b) Histoplasma

INVESTIGATING SUSPECTED LAXATIVE ABUSE
1. ↓ Serum K+
2. + KOH test
3. + Urinary Phenolphthalein
4. **Melanosis coli** on endoscopy; barium enema shows a **loss of haustra** (beware, both of these findings can also be seen in Carcinoid syndrome)

BLOODY DIARRHEA—MICROBIOLOGICAL CAUSES ✪
1. Yersinia
2. Entameba histolytica
3. E. Coli 0157H7
4. Shigella (remember! *no* bloody diarrhea in *Salmonella*)
5. Campylobacter jejuni
6. C. diff (if recent Abx)

STRICTURE IN CROHN'S DISEASE—DDX
1. Adhesions from prior surgeries
2. Carcinoma
3. Inflammatory stenosis
4. Ischemic fibrosis
5. Pericolic abscess
6. Transient bowel spasm

MANAGEMENT OF DES (Diffuse Esophageal Spasm) (AKA 'nutcracker' esophagus)
1. Avoid stress and cold or hot liquids, all of which exacerbate the episodes of chest pain.
2. Be sure you've ruled out CAD/gallstones/PUD
3. Nifedipine
4. Nitrates

SCLERODERMA ✪
1. Progressive dysphagia to solids & liquids
2. Look for these on the UGI:
   a) **Common E-G tube**
   b) **Pseudoobstruction**
   c) **Wide-mouthed jejunal diverticula**
3. Motility studies show aperistalsis in the body of the esophagus; LES incompetence→ severe reflux.

HEMOCHROMATOSIS ✪
1. A disorder of Fe metabolism and Fe overload, with subsequent Fe deposition in multiple organs (heart, pancreas, gonads, joints, skin)
2. Transferrin saturation usually >90%
3. Phlebotomize to keep Hgb<10, male ferritin <350, female ferritin< 200. This approach prevents the development of liver disease, cardiac disease, or skin bronzing.
4. *Arthropathy* and *hypogonadism* and *cirrhosis* are the irreversible complications; the insulin requirement in established diabetics is rarely eliminated, although control may improve.
5. Re: ↑ risk of hepatoma in patients with cirrhosis.

WILSON'S DISEASE ✪
1. Autosomal dominant disease, where, **secondary to defective copper metabolism *in the liver*, it is deposited in a variety of tissues** (as opposed to hemochromatosis, which is 2° to ↑Fe *absorption*→mechanism unknown)—both, however, give a transaminitis.
2. Definitely must know what's ↑ and what's ↓:
   a) Copper in the serum, urine, and liver are **ALL INCREASED**
   b) **DECREASED serum ceruloplasmin** (carrier protein for Cu) <200. In 5%, though, >200.
3. **KAISER-FLEISCHER RINGS** (a brownish pigmented ring at the edge of the cornea)
4. *Neurologic signs*→eg flapping tremor; chorea; rigidity; dysarthria; parkinsonism; abnl gait
5. **HEMOLYTIC ANEMIA**
6. Treatment:
   a) Lifelong oral chelation with **penicillamine**, which ↑s urinary Cu excretion;
   b) Oral zinc or potassium salts to ↓ absorption.

✪ DRUG-INDUCED HEPATIC DISEASE:

Viral Hepatitis	Halothane; INH; ketoconazole
Reye's syndrome	ASA; valproate
Steatosis	TCN; AZT; valproic acid
Crytogenic cirrhosis	Long-term MTX; amiodarone; ↑VitA; vinyl chloride
Primary Biliary Cirrhosis	Chlorpromazine (Thorazine®)
Chronic Active Hepatitis (CAH)	Methyldopa; INH; nitrofurantoin; dantrolene
Budd-Chiari Syndrome	Synthetic estrogens
Granulomatous (hypersensitivity) hep.	Allopurinol
Alcoholic liver disease mimicked by…	Amiodarone
Acute Hepatitis	Acetaminophen (SGOT>4000)—may occur at relatively low doses in alcoholics
Massive ischemic necrosis	Cocaine
Peliosis Hepatis	Androgenic steroids; OCPs
Angiosarcoma	Vinyl chloride; thoratrast; anabolic steroids
Cholestatic Hepatitis	Amoxicillen-clavulinate; oral contraceptive pills

INFECTIOUS DIARRHEA—INDICATIONS FOR ANTIBIOTICS
1. Always
   a. Giardiasis→Flagyl®
   b. Amebiasis—if symptomatic→Flagyl®
   c. Shigella—positive blood culture or severe dysentery only→Cipro®
2. Usually
   a. Pseudomembranous colitis (re: ampicillen; clindamycin; lincamycin
   b. predispose)→PO Flagyl® or Vanco
3. Occasionally
   a. Campylobacter enterocolitis→Erythromycin
   b. Traveler's diarrhea (E. Coli)

INDICATIONS FOR COLECTOMY IN ULCERATIVE COLITIS

1. Acute complications

2. Development of carcinoma (colonic or cholangiocarcinoma)

3. Intractable pararectal or extraintestinal complications

4. Severe colitis with failure to stabilize on medical regimen

5. Severe dysplasia (remember, these patients must receive frequent periodic monitoring with colonoscopy and biopsy)

6. Unacceptable treatment side effects

RESPONSE OF COMPLICATIONS OF ULCERATIVE COLITIS TO <u>COLECTOMY</u> ✪:

1. *Positive Response*
   i)   **P** eripheral arthropathy (don't confuse with hemochromatosis, where treatment *does not* improve the arthropathy)
   ii) **P** yoderma gangrenosum (and the other noteworthy dermatologic manifestation, erythema nodosum)
   iii) **P** ara-rectal disease

2. *Unresponsive*
   i)   **S** pondilitis, Ankylosing (Remember, 'S' for Stays the same!)
   ii) **S** clerosing cholangitis   (Remember, 'S' for Stays the same!)

GUT ENDOCRINE TUMORS

SOMATOSTATINOMA
1. *The delta cells of the <u>pancreas</u> → somatostatin. Stimulates gastric emptying, but inhibits almost everything else* (gastric acid/pepsin secretion; pancreatic and biliary secretions; celiac blood flow; release of GH, TSH, insulin, glucagon, gastrin, and secretin)
2. Used successfully in VIPoma diarrhea control; gastrinoma; insulinoma; glucagonoma; used also in GI hemorrhage and pancreatitis.

VIPoma (vip=vasoactive intestinal peptide)
1. Primary tumor usually pancreatic, producing ↑VIP, resulting in…
2. *Profuse, watery diarrhea* (**secretory** diarrhea—frequently nocturnal or fasting), dehydration, ↓K+
3. Other clinical…
   a) Colicky abdominal pain ("**pancreatic** cholera")
   b) Achlorhydria
   c) Flushing, Hypotension
   d) Hypercalcemia (± MEN I)
4. Treatment: Somatostatin drug of choice for symptom control

GLUCAGONOMA
1. Primary *α-cell <u>pancreatic</u> tumor→glucagon excess.*
2. Present with diarrhea (no steatorrhea), stomatitis, glossitis, thromboembolism, *<u>necrolytic migratory erythema</u>* (transient bullous or crusting rash, often involving perineum and leaving residual pigmentation)
3. *Glucose intolerance* (re, you give glucagon IM when patient is hypoglycemic and unresponsive in order to bring up their sugar)
4. ↓cholesterol; spontaneous, asymptomatic remissions common.
5. Tx: Somatostatin for the diarrhea, anticoagulants for any thromboses, insulin if required.

GASTROENTEROLOGY

GASTRINOMA

1. *Ectopic G-cell tumor, usually found in <u>pancreatic</u> body/tail.*
2. 50% have associated MEN I
3. 50% present with diarrhea or steatorrhea
4. 95% present with duodenal ulceration, classically
    a) Young patient without risk factors (unless MEN I)
    b) Multiple, large, deep ulcers
    c) Ectopic location
    d) May be associated with pyloric stenosis or esophageal stricture
    e) Require very high doses of proton-pump inhibitors, such as omeprazole.
    f) Pancreatic enzyme supplements may be necessary for steatorrhea
    g) Cholestyramine may be helpful in diarrhea

ZOLLINGER-ELLISON SYNDROME

1. *Gastrinoma* → usually ectopic G cell hypersecretion
2. Tumor usually located in the *pancreatic head*
3. 2/3rds of them are malignant
4. ¼ of them have MEN I
5. 90-95% develop *ulceration*; 75% involve the *duodenal bulb* (a single duodenal ulceration is the most common radiographic finding in ZES)
6. Suspect in: *recurrent* duodenal ulcers; PUD that is *poorly responsive* to the usual treatment; ulcers in patients with stigmata of *MEN I*; and *post-bulbar or multiple* ulcers; hypertrophied gastric rugae.
7. Diarrhea (from large amounts of HCL secreted→ >15 meq/h) is present in 1/3 and may precede the ulcer symptoms.
8. Steatorrhea (from inactivation of pancreatic lipase and precipitation of bile salts) may be seen.
9. Prominent gastric folds seen on barium
10. Serum *<u>fasting gastrin level (>1200</u>* pg/ml + low pH) is the most sensitive and specific test (although hypergastrinemia is noted in several other disorders, including: pernicious anemia and chronic atrophic gastritis)
11. *<u>Secretin test</u>*→ normal gastrin (↓) response in patients with simple duodenal ulcer (secretin normally inhibits gastrin); *paradoxical ↑ in gastrin response with ZES*.
12. Localization intraop can be difficult. Selective arteriograms see 1/3 of them, as do CT scans.
13. H2-receptor blockers, proton pump inhibitors, somatostatin, and surgery are the tx available.
14. 20-25% of gastrinomas are surgically resectable
15. Prognosis: **if** resection is curative→ can expect a normal life expectancy; **if not**→ average life expectancy is only 2 years.

CARCINOID SYNDROME—CLINICAL PRESENTATION—"*F.A.C.A.D.E.S.*"

1. **F** lushing; facial edema
2. **A** sthma (wheezing)
3. **C** or Pulmonale
4. **A** scites
5. **D** iarrhea
6. **E** ndocardial fibrosis

7. **S** omatostatin (Octreotide) effective for flushing, diarrhea, carcinoid crisis); **S** econdaries in or beyond the liver produce the *symptoms (for "syndrome", there must be hepatic metastasis present)*

    Remember…
- Order a *urinary 5-HIAA* levels (a serotonin metabolite) for diagnosis
- Vital signs: ↑Temp, ↓BP (2° to vasodilatation), ↑Pulse
- Re: 90% of the tumors are in the terminal ileum
- ***If the gut is normal, look for tumor in the bronchus or gonads***
- In referral centers, this is the #1 cause of watery diarrhea
  - --Proctoscopy reveals *melanosis coli and absent haustra* (similar proctoscopy to laxative abuse)

STRESS ULCERS
1. Cushing's and Curling's ulcers
2. **Curling's ulcers** follow *burns* (might think: "Curling iron")
3. **Cushing's ulcers** are seen in 50-75 % of *head injuries* (might remember: the injury could have been prevented had they been wearing their helmet, or "cushion")
4. Bleeding occurs in 10-20% from 3-7 days following the stress (trauma, stress, illness, burns, etc) if no prophylactic regimen is instituted (Sucralfate; H_2 blockers)

BARRETT'S ESOPHAGUS
1. Columnar-lined esophageal metaplasia; complication of chronic reflux
2. Found in 10% of biopsies for esophagitis
3. Found in 40% of patients with chronic peptic strictures
4. Associated with a 30x ↑ risk of esophageal **adenoca** (along with alcohol, smoking, lye stricture, smoked foods, achalasia, Plummer-Vinson syndrome; tylosis); re: esophageal ca (in general):
   - Male: Female ratio = 4:1
   - 50% are squamous; 50% are adenoca.
   - Usually unresectable; treatment is predominantly palliative
5. Endoscopic surveillance important: If multiple foci of high-grade dysplasia develop, resection may be indicated.
6. 30% of patients presenting with carcinoma in Barrett's have no prior history of reflux.

RECOMMENDATIONS BY LEVEL OF DYSPLASIA ON ENDOSCOPY

No dysplasia: Repeat endoscopy q2y
PPI (proton pump inhibitor) therapy for symptoms

Low-grade dysplasia: Intensive PPI therapy
Repeat endoscopy @ 8wk. If dysplasia found, repeat endoscopy every 6 mo until 2 consecutive exams show no dysplasia, then q year

High-grade dysplasia: Confirm dx with another pathologist
Intensive PPI therapy
Esophagectomy or endoscopic ablation therapy

PLUMMER-VINSON SYNDROME

1. Hypopharyngeal webs (esophageal stricture)
2. Fe deficiency anemia
3. Classically middle-aged women
4. 15% chance of developing oropharyngeal or esophageal ca

DYSPHAGIA

1. Intermittent dysphagia is caused by rings/webs/motility disorders.
2. 2 causes: **mechanical (obstruction) vs. functional (motility)**
3. Diagnosis by **history** can usually be had by getting this information on the dysphagia
   a) Is it to solids or both solids and liquids?
   b) Progressive or intermittent?
   c) Is there associated heartburn?
4. **Schatski's ring** is a *ring at the level of the LES that can present with episodic dysphagia to solid food at diameters less than 1.3cm*
5. **Zenker's diverticulum**
   a) Aka "crycopharyngeal diverticulum"
   b) Cliinical: **halitosis, regurgitation, dysphagia, chronic cough, recurrent pneumonia**.
   c) Treatment is surgical excision of the diverticulum

✪ UNDERSTANDING DYSPHAGIA BY PRESENTATION:

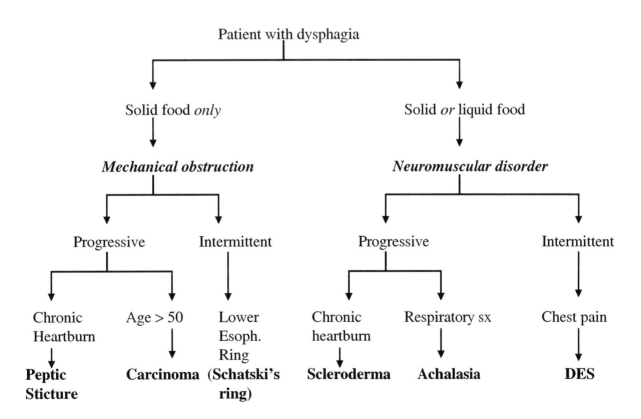

GASTROENTEROLOGY

VERTICAL TRANSMISSION OF HEPATITIS IN PREGNANCY

1. HBV most likely to be transmitted if acquired in the 3rd trimester
2. Neonates at risk should be immediately started on both active and passive immunization; 90% of infected neonates become chronic carriers.
3. Approximately 50% of vertically-infected children ultimately die of cirrhosis or hepatoma

HEPATIC ADENOMAS IN OCP USE (OR PREGNANCY)...
   ✪ May present with **acute RUQ pain and hemodynamic compromise 2° to bleeding/ rupture**.

✪ GLUTEN-SENSITIVE ENTEROPATHY (aka **CELIAC SPRUE**, or "sprue", as opposed to "tropical sprue")
1. AutoAbs may be seen: *+ Anti-endomysial Ab; + Anti-gliadin Ab; + Anti-reticulin Ab*
2. Persistent non-specific GI upset
3. *Fe deficiency anemia*
4. Steatorrhea
5. Growth retardation
6. Osteomalacia($2°$ to ↓ vit D)
7. *Dermatitis Herpetiformis*—classic rash of celiac disease
8. Proctalgia fugax
9. *Remember, the most definitive diagnosis is had by noting symptomatic resolution on a gluten-free diet* (avoid→wheat, rye, barley, oats, malt; may have→ rice, corn, soybean)
10. Howell-Jolly bodies on peripheral blood smear may be seen
11. ↓ RBC folate seen in 70%

INFECTIONS OF THE ESOPHAGUS

1. Candida, HSV, and CMV are the most important causes of odynophagia
2. CMV: severe inflammation with large ulcers
3. HSV: Barium and EGD show small, discrete ulcers; Biopsy shows intranuclear inclusions (Cowdry bodies)

COMPLICATIONS OF GASTRECTOMY-*6 D'S*: (Remember botulism has 6 D's too! --see section on "Toxigenic Diarrheas")
   D umping
   D iarrhea
   D izziness
   D ysphagia
   D eficiencies (vitamins, Fe)
   D istension after eating

BLIND-(or "Stagnant"-) LOOP SYNDROME —"*SALAD*":

S teatorrhea
A nemia
L oss of weight
A bdominal pains
D eficiencies of vitamins

- *Mechanism of BLIND-LOOP SYNDROME*→Bacterial overgrowth occurs in the **afferent loop** and causes malabsorption (as bile salts are deconjugated) and **megaloblastic anemia** as bacteria consume B12; ↓**B12** may also be 2° to loss of Intrinsic Factor that occurs with gastrectomy. Treatment is to convert the Bilroth II→Bilroth I or Roux-en-Y. This **syndrome should not be confused for "afferent loop syndrome"**, which is another complication of Bilroth II that occurs earlier than blind loop syndrome and results, not from bacterial overgrowth complications, but from partial obstruction of the afferent loop.

BRIEF SYNOPSIS OF THE TREATMENTS FOR MALABSORPTION DISORDERS:

Diagnosis	Treatment
Abetalipoproteinemia	Low-fat diet; fat-soluble vitamins
Bacterial overgrowth	Antibiotics
Crohn's disease	5-ASA, steroids
Intestinal infection with:	
Giardia lamblia	Metronidazole
Isospora belli	TMP/SMX
Strongyloides stercoralis	Thiabendazole
Lactase deficiency (Lactose intolerance)	Lactase supplementation
Lymphangiectasia	Address the causative disease
Pancreatic insufficiency	Pancreatic enzyme supplements
Short-gut syndrome	Medium-chain triglycerides, low-oxalate diet, parenteral nutrition as appropriate
Sprue Celiac Tropical	Gluten-free diet B12, folate, TCN
Whipple's disease	Initial IV tx then PO x 1year with Bactrim-ds bid or Cefixime 400 qd(see "Whipple's" below)

INITIAL SCREENING TESTS FOR SUSPECTED MALABSORPTION
Stool Tests
1. 72h quantitative fecal fat
2. O&P

Blood Tests
1. Alkaline phosphatase
2. Blood levels of vitamin B12, folate, vitamin D and K, Calcium, carotene
3. CBC
4. Serum protein
5. Thyroid function

✪ DIAGNOSTIC APPROACH TO MALABSORPTION:

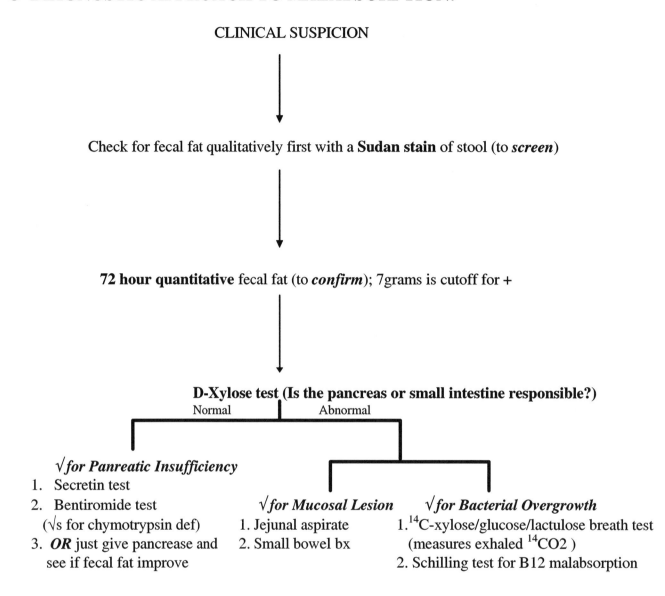

CLINICAL SUSPICION

Check for fecal fat qualitatively first with a **Sudan stain** of stool (to *screen*)

72 hour quantitative fecal fat (to *confirm*); 7grams is cutoff for +

D-Xylose test (Is the pancreas or small intestine responsible?)

Normal   Abnormal

√ for Panreatic Insufficiency
1. Secretin test
2. Bentiromide test
   (√s for chymotrypsin def)
3. **OR** just give pancrease and
   see if fecal fat improve

√ for Mucosal Lesion
1. Jejunal aspirate
2. Small bowel bx

√ for Bacterial Overgrowth
1. ^{14}C-xylose/glucose/lactulose breath test
   (measures exhaled $^{14}CO_2$)
2. Schilling test for B12 malabsorption

IMPORTANT NOTES:

- **D-Xylose test**— A 5-hour urine xylose excretion < 4.5g following ingestion of 25g of D-Xylose indicates mucosal disease or bacterial overgrowth.
- **Secretin test**—Under fluoroscopic guidance, pancreatic secretions are collected in the second part of the duodenum before and after an IV dose of secretin; diagnostic of pancreatic exocrine insufficiency if there is a ↓ in pancreatic fluid output and bicarbonate secretion after secretin; highly sensitive & specific, but invasive and requires excellent patient cooperation. *This ≠ the secretin test in ZES!* (see GI)
- **Bentiromide test** (a synthetic peptide attached to PABA)—Chymotryspin cleaves the two and you check levels of arylamine (a biproduct of PABA) in the urine; low levels are diagnostic of panc insufficiency.
- ^{14}**C-xylose breath test**—Elevated levels indicate bacterial overgrowth. *This ≠ the D-Xylose test!*

EXTRAGASTROINTESTINAL SIGNS IN MALABSORPTION (Mayo IMBR):

EXTRA-GI SYMPTOM	RESULT OF
Muscle wasting, edema	↓Protein absorption
Paresthesias, tetany	↓Vit D and Ca absorption
Bone pain	↓Ca absorption
Muscle cramps; weakness	↓ K+
Easy bruising, petechiae	↓ Vit K absorption
Hyperkeratosis, night blindness	↓ Vit A absorption
Pallor	↓ Vit B12, folate, or Fe absorption
Glossitis, stomatitis, cheilosis	↓ Vit B12, folate, or Fe absorption
Acrodermatitis	↓ Zinc absorption

BILE ACID MALAPSORPTION

1. Diarrhea following ileal disease or resection
2. If the disease/resection is <100 cm→ treatment is **cholestyramine**
3. If the disease/resection is > 100cm→ treatment is **medium chain triglycerides** with a low fat diet

MECKEL'S DIVERTICULUM—*RULE OF 2'S*:

- ◆ 2:1 Male: Female ratio
- ◆ 2 complications: hemorrhage and perforation
- ◆ 2 types of ectopic tissue: gastric and pancreatic
- ◆ Confused with 2 other problems: ulcers and appendix
- ◆ 2% incidence on autopsies (i.e. affects 2% of population)
- ◆ Usually occurs within 2 feet of the ileocecal valve
- ◆ Usually presents within the first 2 years of life
- ◆ Usually about 2 inches in length

CAUSES OF BILIARY TRACT OBSTRUCTION—*"S EX CAN B SC ARY"*

S tones

Ex trinsic compression

Can cer

B lood (hematobilia)

SC lerosing Cholangitis

CLINICAL FEATURES OF **ACUTE** PANCREATITIS—"*AMYLASE*"

A cute pain; **A** lcohol is the #1 cause (acute on chronic) and gallstones are #2.

M id-abdominal staining (Grey Turner's and Cullen's signs)—loin and periumbilical respectively

Y ellow (ascites)

L ipase ↑; **L** eft-sided pleural effusion

A mylase ↑ (usu. > 1000)

S entinel loop (**S** mall bowel ileus overlying the pancreatic area)

E mesis and nausea

CLINICAL FEATURES OF **CHRONIC** PANCREATITIS—"**C** *MAIDS*"

(think "Old maid(s)" for chronic)

C alcification, pancreatic; **C** hronic (!)

M alabsorption

A bdominal pain (Alcohol is the #1 cause, similar to AP)

I cterus

D iabetes

S teatorrhea

✪ **POOR PROGNOSTICATORS IN ACUTE PANCREATITIS** (**RANSON'S CRITERIA**)

At Time of Admission or Diagnosis:

1. Age>55yo
2. WBC>16
3. Glucose (serum)>200
4. LDH>250
5. SGOT (ALT) >350

During Initial 48 hours

1. ↓ in Hct >10%
2. Serum Ca <8
3. ↑ in BUN >5
4. Arterial pO2<60
5. Base Deficit >4
6. Estimated fluid sequestration >600 cc

CONDITIONS ASSOCIATED WITH ACUTE PANCREATITIS

1. *Hypertriglyceridemia (Types 1,4,5)*
2. *Hypercalcemia*. If see, R/O:
   a) Multiple myeloma
   b) Hyperparathyroidism
   c) Metastatic Ca.
3. Pancreas divisum--failure of ventral and dorsal pancreas to fuse during organogenesis;
4. *Post-ERCP*

✪ **DRUGS THAT CAUSE PANCREATITIS:** *"PD FAST VET"* (as in "Pretty Fast corVETte"):

P entamidine
D di (didanosine)

F urosemide
A zathioprine
S ulfa
T hiazides

V alproic acid
E strogen
T etracycline

COMPLICATIONS OF ACUTE PANCREATITIS

1. *Phlegmon*—a mass of inflamed pancreatic tissue

2. *Pseudocysts* ✪—**fluid collections—resolve spontaneously most of the time within weeks**

3. *Hypocalcemia* (2° to accumulation/precipatation of calcium salts)

4. *Pancreatic abscess* ✪—**usually occurs 2-4 weeks after the acute episode: see fever; persistent abdominal pain; persistent ↑ amylase. These MUST be drained!**
5. *ARDS*; and left-sided pleural effusion

PANCREATIC CA
1. The 5 year survival rate is < 2%, since most patients present late in the course of their disease. If patients are diagnosed early enough (tumor<2cm; no nodes; no mets)→Whipple procedure.
2. Courvoisier's sign=painless jaundice with a palpable gallbladder→pancreatic ca
3. Trousseau's sign=recurrent migratory thrombophlebitis→associated with pancreatic ca.
4. "Double-duct" sign=obstruction and therefore visible dilatation of both bile and pancreatic ducts, and is secondary to pancreatic ca; a classic presentation.

WHIPPLE'S DISEASE ✪
1. *Diarrhea (malabsorptive)*
2. *Fever*
3. *Lymphadenopathy*
4. *Migratory arthralgias*
5. Neurologic symptoms
6. Causative organism (found in these macrophages) is Tropheryma Whippllii, a gram + bacillus
7. Treatment: *Initial IV*: Ceftriaxone 2.0g bid + Streptomycin 1.0g qd; *then PO Rx for 1 year with either* TMP/SMX-DS bid or Cefixime 400mg PO qd.

✪ CHRONIC GASTRITIS: TYPE A OR B

Type A
1. ***Associated with*** pernicious anemia (think "A" for autoimmune) and gastric carcinoids. ⟷ **Type B** Associated with ***H. Pylori*** (& PUD)
2. ***Body/fundus*** of stomach ⟷ ***Antrum*** of stomach
3. ↑ Serum gastrin ⟷ ***Normal*** serum gastrin

- ***Both*** Types are associated with ***adenocarcinoma***.

H. PYLORI AND PUD

- H. Pylori is responsible for <u>chronic (type B) antral gastritis</u> and accounts for 80% and 90% of <u>gastric and duodenal PUD</u> respectively.

- Eradication of H. Pylori, using various combinations of bismuth, proton pump inhibitor, H2-receptor antagonists and antibiotics ↓ the rate of recurrence of both gastric and duodenal ulcers. (see below)

- H. Pylori can be tested in the gastroenterologist's office using a <u>CLO test</u> on the endoscopy specimen→agar changes color when presented with the urease-splitting organism.

- H. Pylori is also implicated in the etiology of <u>gastric ca.</u>

- Re: duodenal ulcers are 4x more common than gastric ulcers in this country. Recall that gastric ulcers, if > 2.5cm or suspicious in radiologic appearance, require endoscopy with biopsy, as gastric ulcers have an ↑ risk of malignant transformation.

POINTS ON H. PYLORI TESTING

- **The <u>Urease Breath Test</u>.** The UBT employs ^{13}C and ^{14}C-labeled urea to detect **active** H. Pylori infection. ***The test works as follows:*** if the bacteria are present in the stomach, the urease they produce will hydrolyze labeled urea ingested by the patient, resulting in the release of labeled CO_2, which is measured as the patient breaths into a collection device.

- The ^{13}C and ^{14}C UBTs **can also be used to confirm eradication after treatment** (stool testing is another noninvasive method shown to compare will with the breath test). However, ***proper <u>timing is important</u>:*** testing must be done ≥ 2 weeks after cessation of maintenance antisecretory therapy and ≥ 4 weeks after completion of antibiotic therapy (4 weeks post treatment for stool antigen detection). Remember, **antibody testing with ELISA** is less useful in the evaluation of posttreatment response because high levels of antibodies to H. pylori remain for variable and extended periods. However, for an individual more than a year out from therapy, seroconversion is a reliable indicator of successful eradication.

MULTIDRUG TREATMENT REGIMENS FOR ERADICATING H. PYLORI
Bismuth-based
Bismuth + TCN + Metronidazole
Bismuth + Amox + Metronidazole
Bismuth + TCN + Metronidazole + H2 receptor antagonist
Bismuth + Amox + Metronidazole + H2 receptor antagonist
H2 receptor antagonist-based
Ranitidine + Clarithromycin + Metronidazole
Ranitidine + Amox + Metronidazole
PPI-based
PPI + Clarithromycin + Metronidazole
PPI + Amox + Metronidazole
PPI + Bismuth + TCN + Metronidazole
PPI + Bismuth + Amox + Metronidazole

DIARRHEAS

OSMOTIC DIARRHEA

1. Diarrhea stops with fasting
2. Stool has **+ anion gap**
3. Volume<1L/day

SECRETORY DIARRHEA

Diarrhea persists despite NPO
No anion gap
Volume >1L/day

- In acute diarrhea, no evaluation is necessary unless there are bloody stools and Fever or infection is suspected. In these cases, classically at least, antimotility drugs should not be administered.

RIGHT-SIDED DIARRHEA

1. Large stool volume
2. *No* urgency/tenesmus/mucus/blood
3. Anemia, insidious

LEFT-SIDED DIARRHEA

1. Small amounts of stool
2. *May* note: urgency, tenesmus, mucus, or blood
3. Constipation/obstipation; usually presents sooner

- **Chronic diarrhea** lasts ***longer than 4 weeks*** by definition. The #1 cause is IBS. Must r/o Lactose intolerance (lactase deficiency). Be able to ddx organic (e.g. food poisoning) vs. functional (e.g. IBS) diarrheas. Essentially, in **IBS**, there is no weight loss; no blood in stool; so-called "pencil" (thin) stools; chronicity (> 6 mo); small stool quantity; diarrhea occurs primarily in AMs and rarely wakens the patient; significant association of bowel symptoms with level of stress. These are all in contrast to organic diarrheas.

✪ **Key Features of <u>TOXIGENIC</u> Bacterial Diarrheas—<u>*WATERY*</u>; <u>*NO*</u> *fecal leukocytes*…**

Staph aureus	Rapid onset(2-4h) after custard-filled pastries and delicatessen meats.
Clostridium botulinum (botulism)	Neurotoxin interferes with presynaptic ACh release, causing the other 6D's→Dilated fixed pupils; Diplopia; Dysarthria; Dysphagia; Dry tongue; Descending paralysis.
Clostridium perfringes	"Church picnic"/buffet diarrhea; precooked foods; later in onset than Staph aureus
E. Coli, enterotoxigenic	Traveler's diarrhea; Cipro prophylactically; if develops, may take Cipro bid for 3 days, although usually self-limiting.
Vibrio cholerae	The only toxigenic bacterial diarrhea where Abx clearly ↓ disease duration (TCN)
B. Cereus	Fried rice in oriental restaurants

✪ **Key Features of some <u>INVASIVE</u> Bacterial Diarrheas—*Fever; BLOODY stools; and + fecal leukocytes*…**

Salmonella	**No antibiotics, unless** + blood culture; also do **not** see bloody diarrhea with Salmonella (the exception); eggs/poultry/fecal-oral route
Vibrio parahemolyticus	Undercooked shellfish
Yersinia enterocolytica	DDx includes AP and Crohn's disease; dairy products
E. Coli 0157H7 (enterhemorrhagic E. Coli)	**No** fever here; tainted beef/milk→HUS.
Vibrio vulnificus (noncholera)	Skin/muscle inflammation/infection after exposure to seawater or cleaning fish; & septicemia/necrotizingvasculitis/gangrene/ shock after ingesting raw oysters.
Others: Shigella; Campylobacter (below)	

CAMPYLOBACTER JEJUNI ENTERITIS

1. Remember the association with ***Guillain-Barre Syndrome*** (ascending paralysis— as opposed to the descending paralysis of botulism, above)

2. More common cause of enteritis than Salmonella or Shigella.

3. Bloody diarrhea/toxic megacolon/HLA B27+ reactive athritis are all potential complications and may therefore resemble Ulcerative Colitis.

4. Treatment is Erythromycin.

BLOODY DIARRHEA WITHOUT VOMITING…

1. Campylobacter jejuni

2. Amebiasis

SYSTEMIC MASTOCYTOSIS

1. 2° to proliferation of mast cells in numerous organs
2. ↑histamine released; 50% of patients have GI symptoms, such as PUD and diarrhea
3. *Urticaria pigmentosa*
4. *"Bath pruritis" (similar to P. Vera)*

✪ AMYLOIDOSIS (*"AMY gives her P's TLC"*)

1. Macroglossia (**T**ongue)
2. Hepatomegaly (**L**iver)
3. Cardiomegaly (**C**ardiac)
4. **P**roteinuria
5. **P**eripheral neuropathy
6. **P**alpable **P**urpura
7. **P**inch (post-traumatic) or **P**eriorbital ecchymoses **P**ost-**P**roctoscopy
8. GI symptoms, such as motility disorders and malabsorption, are 2° to amyloid infiltration into muscle and nerve.
9. Skin-**P**opping in type B ("AA"), not type A ("AL") phenotype
10. Fat and rectal biopsies very useful in diagnosis.

PSEUDO-OBSTRUCTION

1. Acute intestinal pseudoobstruction is often referred to as *Ogilvie's syndrome*.
2. Clinical findings of mechanical obstruction but without occlusion of the lumen; usu. the colon
3. *Abnormal esophageal motility* in most patients
4. *Steatorrhea* (caused by bacterial overgrowth)
5. *2° causes include→* amyloidosis, Parkinson's disease, myxedema, hypoparathyroidism, L-Dopa, TCA's, clonidine, phenothiazines, and narcotics.

ULCERATIVE COLITIS AND CROHN'S DISEASE

1. UC involves the **colorectal intestine**
   ♦ While Crohn's may involve **any** part of the intestinal tract (other than the rectum—"rectal sparing"), and is associated with **perianal** disease (e.g.strictures/fistulas/abscesses→Flagyl)
2. UC has frequent, bloody BMs, while Crohn's has more abdominal pain, fewer BMs, and less bleeding.

3. UC may have **pseudopolyps and crypt abscesses. Toxic megacolon** is a complication of particular concern in UC, and opiates may precipitate (just as anti-motility drugs can in patients with hematochezia and fever, e.g. many of the invasive bacterial diarrheas)

4. **Colonoscopy is contraindicated in acute UC due to the ↑ risk of perforation.**

5. ✪ Among the extraintestinal manifestations: *the severity of joint and skin disease mirrors the severity of colitis.* On the other hand, ankylosing spondylitis and sacroiliitis do not mirror the colitis.

6. Remember, **C** rohn's→ Calcium oxalate stones **(C→C)**
   U C   → Uric acid stones   **(U→U)**

7. Colectomy is curative in UC

8. **Common Medications in UC (by location):**

   Mesalamine: 1) RowASA suppository/enema for relief of ***proctitis***
                   2) PentASA for relief of ***small bowel*** inflammatory disease; work by releasing ASA into small bowel
                   3) ASAcol best choice for ***terminal ileum*** disease.

   Olsalazine and Sulfasalazine: for ***colonic*** disease; also work by releasing ASA into the colon

9. **Common Medications for Crohn's (by location):**

   Metronidazole→for ***perianal*** disease; may switch from sulfasalazine → metronidazole, but not vise versa.

♦   *Note, sulfasalazine is important in maintaining remission in UC only, not Crohn's. It is used for active disease in Crohn's.*

DRUGS TO TREAT IBD (by situation)	
Situation	*Commonly Used Options*
ULCERATIVE COLITIS	
Proctitis, distal colitis	Topical 5-ASA, topical hydrocortisone, PO 5-ASA
Mild to moderate	Oral 5-ASA, oral steroids
Severe	Oral or IV steroids, IV cyclosporine
Refractory disease or steroid dependent	Addition of 6-mercaptopurine or azathioprine
Maintenance of remission	*Oral sulfasalazine*, oral 5-ASA, topical 5-ASA for distal disease
CROHN'S DISEASE	
Mild to moderate	Oral 5-ASA, oral steroids, metronidazole
Severe	Parenteral steroids
Perianal disease	Metronidazole, Ciprofloxacin, addition of 6-MP or azathioprine to standard therapy
Refractory disease, steroid-dependent, or fistulas	Add 6-MP or Azathioprine to standard tx or MTX
Maintenance of remission	*5-ASA, mesalamine (5-aminosalicylic acid)*

GASTROENTEROLOGY

✪ GI DISEASE IN AIDS

1. HSV, CMV, and Candida esophagitis
2. **Histoplasma capsulatum**—colonic involvement; diagnosis by culture; Treatment is ampho or itraconazole
3. **MAI** (mycobacterium avium intracellulare) can cause a voluminous diarrhea and is often associated with additional fever, abdominal pain, and weight loss.
4. **Cryptosporidium**—Voluminous, watery diarrhea. In immunocompromised hosts, especially those with AIDS, diarrhea can be chronic, persistent, and remarkably profuse, causing clinically significant fluid and electrolyte depletion. Stool volumes may range from 1 to 25 L/d.no therapy *proven* efficacious, although in AIDS patients may try treating with paromomycin.
5. **Microsporidia**— Affects the small intestine, causing diarrhea; albendazole is the primary treatment of choice.
6. **Isospora belli**- Diagnosis via oval oocysts in the stool seen with modified Kinyoun acid-fast stain. Primary treatment choice is TMP-SMX (160/800 mg qid for 10 days and then bid for 3 weeks) for treatment.
7. **Entameba histolytica**→Metronidazole; see amebiasis.
8. **Giardia lamblia**→Prominent early symptoms include diarrhea, abdominal pain, bloating, belching, flatus, nausea, and vomiting. Although diarrhea is common, upper intestinal manifestations such as nausea, vomiting, bloating, and abdominal pain may predominate. Associated with camping trips; "white-water rafting"; questions involving "Venezuela"(!); treatment is metronidazole
9. **Cyclospora**--Some patients may harbor the infection without symptoms, but many with cyclosporiasis have diarrhea, flulike symptoms, and flatulence and burping. The diagnosis can be made by detection of spherical 8- to 10-um oocysts in the stool. These refractile oocysts are variably acid-fast and are fluorescent when viewed with ultraviolet light microscopy.
10. **Blastocystis hominis**→ Role as a pathogen is controversial; no controlled rx trials
11. Remember also: When see **Hairy Leukoplakia**→must R/O HIV
12. In **CMV** infection, viremia does not necessarily correlate with organ involvment; therefore, cultures are often of no use in this setting.

✪ ACUTE MESENTERIC ISCHEMIA

1. Usually 2° to *Afib or h/o heart disease*→emboli to the SMA (superior mesenteric artery)→ ischemia→gangrene; may also be 2° to poor perfusion at so-called "watershed" area of intestine.

2. Radiography may show gas in the portal vein; "***thumbprinting***" (2° thick, edematous bowel wall); A/F levels may be seen

3. *Severe abdominal pain* ("out of proportion to the exam") ± shock

4. ↑Anion Gap 2° to lactic acidosis; ↑WBC

5. High mortality

6. **Immediate surgical resection** of the diseased bowel is the treatment.

AMEBIC COLITIS

1. Bloody diarrhea with Fever, tenesmus, and abdominal cramps.
2. Proctoscopy shows discrete ulcers.
3. Concentric narrowing of the cecum 90% of the time.
4. Treatment is metronidazole.

PEARL: *If you're presented with a case of Strep Bovis endocarditis, √ the colon for diverticulosis or colon ca !* ✪

PARACENTESIS:

Transudates *(Protein <2.5g/dl)*	**EXudates** *(Protein > 2.5 g/dl, i.e. "EXceeds")*
CHF/cirrhosis/nephrosis	TB (infEXtion)
Portal HTN	Fungal (infEXtion)
↓Albumin	SBP (infEXtion)
Meig's Syndrome	Cancers (e.g. hepatoma; mesothelioma; mets; ovarian) ("My EX"!

ALBUMIN GRADIENT

✪ Albumin gradient = Serum albumin-Ascites albumin

✪ If this **gradient >1.1 g/dl**→almost always indicative of **portal HTN**, which β-blockers, like *propranolol* can treat to ↓ the risk of variceal bleeding

---

SBP (SPONTANEOUS BACTERIAL PERITONITIS)

1. Is exactly that, and nearly always involves a single organism
2. Fever/abdominal pain and tenderness/ascites
3. ✪ Check the cell count of the ascitic fluid: **PMNs→ usually > 250 (and WBC > 500)**; often culture negative, so don't necessarily rely on the culture, and **when you do culture→innoculate bottles at bedside! Instead, If see ↑PMNs and suspect clinically→start patient on a 3rd generation cephalosporin.**
4. 10-20% of cirrhotic patients develop SBP

HEPATORENAL SYNDROME

1. ARF with normal tubular function in a patient with cirrhosis.
2. Carries a ***high mortality***
3. Can be difficult to distinguish from prerenal failure
4. ***Aggressive diuresis in a cirrhotic can precipitate.***
5. Supportive treatment.

GASTROENTEROLOGY

⊗ **REVISED ACS Guidelines For SCREENING And Surveillance For COLORECTAL POLYPS/CA**

Risk Category	Recommendation[1]	Age to Begin	Interval
Average Risk			
Patients ≥ 50 yo not in any of the categories below	One of the following: 1. FOBT plus FS[2]; or 2. TCE[3]	Age 50	1. FOBT every year and FS q5y 2. Colo q10y or DCBE q5-10y
Moderate Risk			
Single small (<1cm) adenomatous polyps	Colonoscopy	At the time of initial polyp diagnosis	TCE within 3y after initial polypectomy; if normal, as per average recommendations (above)
Large (≥1 cm) or multiple adenomatous polyps of any size	Colonoscopy	At the time of initial polyp diagnosis	TCE within 3y after initial polypectomy; if normal, TCE q5y
Personal h/o curative-intent resection of colorectal ca	TCE[4]	Within 1y after resection	If normal, TCE in 3y; If still normal, TCE q5y
Colorectal ca or adenomatous polyps in 1st degree relative <60 or in 2 1st degree relatives of any age	TCE	Age 40, or 10y before the youngest case in the family, whichever is earlier	Q5y
Colorectal ca in other relatives (not included above)	As per average-risk recommendations (above); may consider screening before 50yo		
High Risk			
Family h/o adenomatous polyps	Early surveillance with endoscopy, counseling to consider genetic testing, and rferral to a specialty center	Puberty	If genetic test is +, or polyposis is confirmed, consider colectomy; otherwise, endoscopy q1-2y
Family h/o HNPCC	Colonoscopy and counseling to consider genetic testing	Age 21	If genetic test is + , or if patient has not had genetic testing, colonoscopy q2y until age 40, and then q year
IBD	Colonoscopies with biopsies for dysplasia	8 years after the start of pancolitis; 12-15 y after the start of L-sided colitis	Q1-2 y

DCBE=double-contrast barium enema; **FOBT** = fecal occult blood test; **FS** = flex sig; **TCE** = total colon examination
1. Digital rectal exam should be done at the time of each flex sig, colonoscopy, or DCBE.
2. Annual FOBT has been shown to reduce mortality from colorectal ca, so it is preferable to no screening.
3. TCE includes either DCBE or TCE.
4. This assumes that a perioperative TCE was done.

OVERVIEW OF COLONIC POLYP PATHOLOGY

1. **Hyperplastic**—these are benign

2. **Adenomatous**
   a) *Villous*—**the real "villains", i.e. carry a greater risk of malignant transformation** (3 times that of tubular)
   b) *Tubular*—much smaller risk of transformation
   c) *Tubulovillous*—halfway in between the two in risk of transformation.

The likelihood that any polypoid lesion in the large bowel contains invasive cancer is *related to the size* of the polyp, being **negligible (<2 percent) in lesions smaller than 1.5 cm**, **intermediate (2 to 10 percent) in lesions 1.5 to 2.5 cm in size**, and **substantial (10 percent) in lesions larger than 2.5 cm**.

✪ *Remember*, **PEUTZ-JEGHERS is a polyposis syndrome** where you see hamartomas of the small intestine and hyperpigmented lesions of mouth/hands/feet. *Remember, these are hamartomas (not adenomas as with most other heritable GI polyposis syndromes), and the malignant potential is PRESENT, BUT QUITE LOW.*

6. INFECTIOUS DISEASE & HIV

VIRAL DISEASES

THE WEST NILE-LIKE VIRUS

♦ A mosquito-borne virus which can cause encephalitis or meningitis
♦ It is spread to humans by the bite of a mosquito that becomes infected when feeding on infected birds.
♦ The virus cannot spread directly from person to person and there is no evidence that a person can get the virus from handling an infected bird.
♦ The incubation period in humans is 5-15 days
♦ Most infections are mild. Symptoms include fever, H/A, and myalgias, often with a skin rash, and lymphadenopathy.
♦ More severe infections may be marked by H/A, high fever, neck stiffness, stupor, disorientation, coma, tremors, convulsions, muscle weakness, paralysis, and rarely, death
♦ Therapy is supportive, as there is no directed therapy.

✪ EBV and INFECTIOUS MONO

1. Look for '**atypical lymphocytes**' on exam
2. Symptoms: fever, fatigue
3. Signs: **splenomegaly**; + LN; exudative pharyngitis
4. Official clinical 'triad' is → 1) Fever; 2) pharyngitis; and 3) cervical lymphadenopathy
5. Lab: ↑**LFT's** (in 80-90%); **+ Monospot** (in 90%); IgM Ab to the VCA (viral capsid Ag) of EBV
6. **If Ampicillen is given, a rash usually always develops.**
7. EBV is also associated with Hodgkin's/B-cell/Burkitt's lymphomas; and nasopharyngeal ca.

Remember, **EBV and CMV** mononucleosis syndromes can look similar clinically. To r/o EBV, √ VCA IgM. To r/o CMV, √ CMV IgM. Note that 'atypical lymphocytes' may be seen in either EBV, CMV, or Toxo, all of which give mono-like syndromes.

CMV

1. Causes a **heterophile-negative** (negative Monospot) mononucleosis syndrome
2. Otherwise it is a fairly benign virus in immunocompetent individuals.
3. CMV is **transmitted via granulocytes**, which harbor the virus. Thus, in immunosuppressed individuals, blood products often require a "Leukotrap" or WBC filter to prevent CMV transmission.

4. In *AIDS and transplant patients, CMV may cause*…

> a) ✪ <u>Retinitis</u> (so-called '<u>ketchup-and-mustard</u>' or '<u>pizza pie</u>' fundoscopic appearance); patient with AIDS complains of <u>floaters</u>; treatment with <u>Gancyclovir (re: bone marrow suppression)</u> or <u>Foscarnet (re: nephrotoxicity</u>) or Cidovidir.

    b) Encephalitis
    c) Pneumonia (more in transplant patients—mortality 50% in these patients)
    d) Esophagitis
    e) GI ulcers
    f) Adrenalitis

MAKING SENSE OF EBV SEROLOGY IN INFECTIOUS MONONUCLEOSIS

1. <u>EA (antibody to EBV 'Early Antigen')</u>
   a) Appears within 2-3 wk of symptom onset
   b) 'D' (diffuse) component disappears within months and is useful marker of ***current infection*** if EA +
   c) 'R' component may persist for years esp in relapsing disease
2. <u>VCA IgM</u> (i.e. IgM to VCA, or viral capsid antigen)
   a) Tends to parallel heterophile Ab ↑
   b) Usually becomes negative within 3 months of symptom onset
   c) ***Extremely useful in heterophile-negative cases; the best test for confirming acute*** disease
3. <u>Heterophile Antibody</u> (IgM)
   a) Test for acute diseased; commonly ordered
   b) May be give false negatives for up to 1 month after symptom onset
   c) Tedious and expensive
4. EBNA (EBV-associated nuclear Ag)
   a) Indicates ***infected cells harboring viral genome***
   b) Viral Ag detected by immunofluorescence
5. EBNA Antibody (IgG)
   a) Appears late
   b) Indicates ***prior infection***; persists lifelong
6. VCA (viral capsid antibody; IgG)—Positive indicates ***past or present*** infection

VZV (VARICELLA ZOSTER VIRUS)

1. Causes Varicella (chicken pox) and Zoster (shingles)
2. Vesicular lesions follow a dermatomal distribution in Zoster
3. *May disseminate, particularly in immunocompromised patients, to give pneumonitis or encephalitis*.
4. Most common complication→Post-herpetic neuralgia

Patients who have never had chicken pox can get chicken pox by exposure to someone with shingles (***but can't get zoster*** since to contract zoster you have to have had chicken pox, as zoster is a manifestation of reactivation of a previous infection).
Seen diagramatically, this is easily summarized:

Zoster ⟷ Chicken pox, but ***never*** Zoster ⟶ Zoster
(can go either way)

HSV-1 and HSV-2
1. Among **genital** HSV infections, HSV-2 is responsible for 75%; HSV-1 for 25%
2. As for **oral** lesions, the distribution is usually the other way around
3. **HSV-1** is usually responsible for **disseminated** HSV infection
4. Encephalitis shows a predilection for the **temporal lobes**
5. **Herpetic whitlow** is a painful finger infection, usu contracted thru needle sticks.
6. Remember, Dermatitis Herpetiformis is a bullous skin complication related to Celiac Disease (gluten-sensitive enteropathy) and has nothing to do with herpes per se.

HTLV-1
1. Associated with **H**uman **T**-cell Leukemia and **chronic myelopathy** ('tropical spastic paraparesis')
2. Transmitted via STD, blood products, IVDA

PARVOVIRUS B19 ✪
1. **Erythema infectiosum** ('fifth disease', 'slapped-cheek syndrome')
2. Found in patients with **pure red blood cell aplasia**
3. **Anemia** in patients with malignancy (e.g. in ALL)
4. Symmetric **polyarthropathy** in adults
5. Giant pronormoblasts seen on bone marrow exam
6. Respond to IV Immunoglobulin

ROTAVIRUS
1. Watery diarrheal illness of children;
2. Winter;
3. Frequently contracted thru swimming pools;
4. Diagnosis by checking stool for antigen, using ELISA;
5. Treatment is symptomatic

NORWALK VIRUS
1. "Winter vomiting disease" in older children and adults
2. N/Vomiting/watery diarrhea very similar to Rotavirus
3. Mild self-limited illness
4. Treatment is also supportive

ASEPTIC MENINGITIS
1. Many causes, but usually viral
2. Usually self-limited
3. CSF pleocytosis (↑monos), negative bacterial cultures

HPV—CLINICAL ASSOCIATIONS ✪ –*see Dermatology for more re: specific subtypes*
1. Plantar warts
2. Flat warts
3. Skin squamous cell carcinoma in transplant patients
4. Genital warts (condyloma acuminata)
5. Oral leukoplakia
6. Squamous Cell Carcinoma of the Cervical/penile/vulva

PRECURSORS TO INVASIVE CERVICAL CARCINOMA
Low-grade Lesions
√ Cellular changes associated with **HPV** infection
√ Mild dysplasia (CIN I)
High-grade Lesions
√ Moderate dysplasia (CIN 2)
√ Severe dysplasia (CIN 3)
√ Carcinoma-in-situ

INFLUENZA
1. Type A most common
2. Those ≥65yo have by far the highest mortality
3. Strep and Staph can secondarily infect
4. **Amantadine** is only effective vs. Type A and can shorten the course of disease in influenza only if given **within 48 hours** of symptom onset (Amantadine as *TREATMENT*)
5. Amantadine + Vaccine confers ± 95% protection (Amantadine as *PROPHYLAXIS)*
6. Amantadine toxicity = restlessness, insomnia, dizziness, renal
7. The flu vaccine **may in fact be given along with Pneumovax**
8. The following **risk groups** should receive annual vaccine
   a) ≥65
   b) > or < 65 with chronic medical problems, such as cardiopulmonary disorders and DM
   c) Health care personnel
   d) Nursing home residents and residents of other long-term care facilities, as well as their staff
   e) House-hold members of high-risk groups
   f) Healthy pregnant women who will be in their 2nd or 3rd trimesters during the flu season.
   g) HIV and immunocompromised
   h) Anyone who wishes to reduce the likelihood of becoming ill with influenza

9. The **neuraminidase inhibitors, Relenza**® **(zanamivir) and Tamiflu**® **(oseltamivir)** are indicated for uncomplicated acute illness due to influenza in patients who have been symptomatic **for ≤ 2 days**. They are effective vs. both influenza types A and B. Neuraminidase is a viral glycoprotein whose function is to break the bond holding new virus particles to infected cells. Once these bonds are broken, new viruses are free to infect other cells. These inhibitors of neuraminidase, *therefore*, are thought to reduce the spread of the virus. Relenza® is the inhaler. Tamiflu® is the capsule.

RABIES

1. A Virus that spreads along peripheral nerves→CNS
2. Cats, dogs, skunks, foxes, raccoons, bats harbor the virus
3. Consider rabies in cases of myelitis or encephalitis of unclear etiology
4. Diagnostics:
   a) Serum and CSF may be tested for rabies Ab
   b) DFA (Direct Fluorescent Ab) testing of biopsy taken from back of neck may be used to detect rabies Ag
   c) Negri bodies seen on hippocampal biopsy specimen are definitive

✪ **HRIG** (Human Rabies Immune Globulin) **+ vaccine** are useful, **but only if begun before the onset of symptoms.**

RABIES POST-EXPOSURE PROPHYLAXIS ✪ —**Cleansing wound with soap & water shown to be protective in 90% of experimental animals**.

Animal	Evaluation/Disposition of Animal	Recommendation for Prophylaxis
Dogs, cats	Healthy and available for 10d observation → Rabid/suspected rabid → Unknown (escaped) →	Don't start unless animal develops sx, then start HRIG (IgG) + vaccine Immediate vaccination Consult public health officials
Skunks, raccoons, bats, foxes, most carnivores	Regard as rabid	Immediate vaccination
Livestock, rodents, rabbits, squirrels, chipmunks, rats, mice, guinea pigs, hamsters, gerbels	N/A	Almost never require anti-rabies vaccine.

✪ N.B. Half of the **HRIG** dose should be injected directly into the **wound** and the rest in the *gluteal* area.
✪ In adults the **Vaccine** should only be given at the *deltoid* area: re days 0,3,7,14,28

PML (Progressive Multifocal Leukoencephalopathy)

1. A slow virus (a papovavirus)
2. Seen in *AIDS, lymphoma, leukemia,*
3. Affects the CNS white matter in an otherwise non-specific pattern

MEASLES (Rubeola)

1. Prodromal URI symptoms common
2. Oral *Koplik's spots* are seen before the skin rash
3. May cause encephalitis
4. *Staph aureus and H. Flu are the most common 2° bacterial infections*, and are, in fact, more common than 1° measles pneumonia.

RUBELLA

1. **Clinical**: fever, transient erythematous rash, posterior cervical LN, and arthralgia.
2. Pregnant women should not be given the vaccine since may cause congenital defects. Remember, it is a *live* vaccine (refer to section on vaccines later in this chapter)
3. For the same reason, women of child-bearing age should be warned not to become pregnant for 2-3 months following vaccination.

4. ✪ *Rubella titre and pregnancy...*

    a) If indicates immune→no treatment necessary

    b) If shows non-immune→follow patient for evidence of clinical rubella and recheck titre in 2-3 wk→if hasn't ↑d and no clinical signs→no treatment necessary.

    c) If, on the other hand, patient has seroconverted or she shows clinical signs of rubella→a *therapeutic abortion* should be considered

HEPATITIS B POST-EXPOSURE PROPHYLAXIS FOR ADULTS ✪ :

EXPOSED PERSON	Exposure SOURCE		
	HBsAg +	HBsAg -	Status Unknown
Unvaccinated	HBIG + Vaccine	Vaccine	Test source for HBsAg
Vaccinated	If exposed person has anti-HBs ≥10→No tx; If < 10→HBIG + 1 dose of vaccine.	No Tx	If exposed person has anti-HBs ≥10→No tx; If < 10→ 1 dose of vaccine.

HIV

ANTIRETROVIRAL TREATMENT FOR HIV (SANFORD GUIDE)

When should anti-retrovirals be started? → "Rule of 5's":

1. <u>CD4<500; or</u>
2. <u>HIV RNA >5000 copies/ml</u>

TREATMENT REGIMENS/COMBINATIONS:

Nucleoside Reverse-Transcriptase Inhibitors (<u>NRTI</u>), aka 'Nucleoside Analogues':
Group "**A**" drugs
    1. Zidovudine (ZDV or AZT)—Retrovir®
    2. Stavudine (d4T) —Zerit®
Group "**B**" drugs
    1. Didanosine (ddI) —Videx®
    2. Zalcitabine (ddC) —HIVID®
    3. Lamivudine (3TC)—Epivir®

Non- Nucleoside Reverse-Transcriptase Inhibitors (<u>NNRTI</u>):
('Non-Nucleoside Analogues')
    1. Nevirapine (Viramune®)
    2. Delavirdine (Rescriptor®)
    3. Efavirenz (Sustiva®)

Protease Inhibitors (<u>PI</u>)
    1. Saquinavir (Invirase®; Fortovase®)
    2. Indinavir (Crixivan®)
    3. Ritonavir (Norvir®)
    4. Nelfinavir (Viracept®)
    5. Amprenavir (Agenerase®)

- **Most experts recommend initiating triple combinations as follows→2 NRTI's ("A" + "B")** *plus either* **a (NNRTI or PI).**
- **Triple therapy as such is** <u>*also*</u> **recommended for 4 weeks following a needle stick injury from an individual known to be HIV+.**

⇒ *Adding one "A" drug to one "B" drug prevents additive toxicities.*

- **Double combination (esp ZDV + 3TC) in patients with less severe** disease (< 5000 viral copies) has shown complete suppression for up to 1 year in 80%

✪ PROPHYLAXIS VS. <u>FIRST EPISODE</u> OF OPPORTUNISTIC DISEASE IN HIV:

Organism	Indication	Drug of Choice	Alternatives
PCP	CD4 <200 or oropharyngeal candidiasis	Bactrim DS QD Bactrim SS QD	• Dapsone/Pyrimethamine/Leukovorin; • Pentamidine (aerosol) • Atovaquone;
MTB			
INH-Sensitive	• PPD ≥5mm; or • Prior +PPD without Rx; or • Contact with active TB case	INH + B6 Rifampin + Pyrazinamide (PZA)	Rifabutin +/- PZA
INH-Resistant	Same; and High prob of exposure to INH-Resistant TB	Rifampin + PZA	Rifabutin +/- PZA
MDR-TB (INH and Rifampin-Resistant)	Same; plus high prob. of exposure to MDR-TB	see section on MDR-TB	see section on MDR-TB
Toxoplasmosis gondii	IgG Ab to Toxoplasma and CD4<100	Bactrim DS	• Dapsone + Pyramethimine + Leucovorin • Atovaquone ± Pyramethamine + Leucovorin
MAI	CD4<50	Azithromycin; or Clarithromycin	Rifabutin ± Azithromycin
VZV	Significant exposure to chickenpox or shingles for patients who have no history of either condition or, if available, neg VZV Ab	Varicella zoster immune globulin (VZIG) as 5 vials IM given ≤ 96h post-exposure	None
Strep pneumoniae	All patients	Pneumovax	None
Hep A	All susceptible (anti-HAV-negative) patients with chronic Hep C	Hep A vaccine: 2 doses	None
Hep B	All susceptible (anti-HBc-negative) patients	Hep B vaccine: 3 doses	None
Influenza	All patients annually	Whole or split virus as IM	Rimantidine; or Amantadine

✪ IMPORTANT RELATED POINTS:

♦ Prophylaxis should also be considered for persons with CD4 <14% and for persons with a h/o of an AIDS-defining illness.

♦ Remember, *TMP-SMX also* reduces the frequency of *toxoplasmosis*. And vice versa, so that...

♦ ...Patients who are being treated for Toxo with *sulfadiazene-pyrimethamine* are protected against PCP and do not need additional prophylaxis against PCP.

♦ Patients receiving **dapsone** should be *tested for G6PD deficiency*.

♦ *Rifampin should not be administered concurrently with protease inhibitors or nonnucleoside reverse transcriptase inhibitors. Rifabutin is an alternative. Even then, rifabutin should not be given with saquinivir or delavirdine.*

♦ *PCP prophylaxis may be d/c'd if* CD4 ≥200 >3-6 months; *and MAI prophylaxis may be d/c'd when* CD4 >100 >3-6 months with evidence of sustained suppression of HIV plasma RNA for a similar period.

♦ **INDICATIONS FOR <u>STEROIDS</u> WHEN INITIATING TREATMENT FOR PCP:**
    1. PaO2 < 70
    2. A-a gradient > 35

♦ For **PCP**, if the patient is **not acutely ill, is able to take PO meds & PaO2 >70**, treatment recommended is:
    1. Dapsone 100 qd + TMP (no SMX) @ 5mg/kd x 21d ; *OR:*
    2. TMP-SMX-DS 2 tabs tid x 21d

♦ Diagnostic procedure of choice in **<u>PCP</u>** is sputum induction. Send for **<u>silver methenamine stain</u>**. If negative → bronchoscopy.

✪ **Prophylaxis to Prevent <u>RECURRENCES</u> of Opportunistic Dz in HIV after Rx for Acute Dz.**

<u>Organism</u>	<u>Drug of Choice</u>	<u>Alternatives</u>
PCP	Bactrim SS or DS	• Dapsone; *or* • Dapsone + Pyimethamine + Leucovorin; *or* • Aerosolized Pentamidine; *or* • Atovaquone
Toxoplasmosis gondii	Sulfadiazine + Pyrimethamine + Leucovorin	• Clindamycin + Pyrimethamine + Leucovorin; *or* • Atovaquone + Pyrimethamine + Leucovorin
MAI	Clarithromycin + Ethambutol ± Rifabutin	Azithromycin + Ethambutol ± Rifabutin
CMV	Ganciclovir; Foscarnet	Cidofovir + Probenicid; *or* Fomivirsen
Cryptococcus Neoformans	Fluconazole	Ampho B; *or* Itraconazole
Histoplasma Capsulatum	Itraconazole	Ampho B
Coccidioides immitis	Fluconazole	Ampho B
Salmonella species (non-typhi)	Ciprofloxacin	(other active antibiotic ok)
RECOMMENDED ONLY FOR FREQUENT OR SEVERE SUBSEQUENT EPISODES:		
HSV	Acyclovir; or Famciclovir	Valacyclovir
Candida (oropharyngeal; esophageal; or vaginal)	Fluconazole	Itraconazole or ketoconazole

MAI (Mycobacterium Avium Intracellulare)

1. Can cause a voluminous diarrhea

2. Typical presentation includes:
   - **Fever,**
   - **Anemia,**
   - **Abdominal pain**, and
   - **Weight loss.**

3. CD4 count < 50-100

IMPORTANT DRUG-DRUG INTERACTIONS IN PROPHYLAXIS OF OPPORTUNISTIC DISEASE:

Affected Drug	Culprit Drug	Effect	Recommendation
Atovaquone	Rifampin	↓	Avoid this combo or ↑ atovaquone dose
Clarithromycin	Ritonavir	↑	No adjustment necessary if normal renal function; adjust if creat clearance <30
Clarithromycin	Nevirapine	↓	Effect of MAI prophylaxis may be ↓'d, so monitor closely
Ketoconazole	Antacids, didanosine (ddI), H2-receptor antagonists, proton-pump inhibitors	↓ absorption	Avoid using ketoconazole with pH-raising agents or use another antifungal
Quinolone antibiotics	Didanosine, antacids, iron products, calcium products, sucralfate	↓	Give quinolone ≥2h prior
Rifabutin	Fluconazole	↑	Monitor rifabutin toxicity such as uveitis, nausea, & neutropenia
Rifabutin	Efavirenz	↓	↑ Rifabutin dose to 450 mg QD
Rifabutin	Ritonavir, saquinavir, indinavir, nelfinavir, amprenavir, delavirdine	↑	Contraindicated with hard-gel saquinivir and delavirdine; Use ½ dose with indinavir, nelfinavir, amprenavir; Use ¼ dose w/ ritonavir

ADVERSE EFFECTS OF MEDS USED IN HIV OPPORTUNISTIC INFECTIONS:

ADVERSE EFFECTS	MEDICATIONS
Bone marrow suppression	Cidofovir, dapsone, gancicolovir, pyrimethamine, rifabutin, sulfadiazine, TMP-SMX
Diarrhea	Atovaquone, clindamycin
Hepatotoxicity	Clarithromycin, fluconazole, INH, itraconazole, ketoconazole, pyrazinamide, rifabutin, rifampin
Nephrotoxicity	Ampho B, cidofovir, foscarnet, pentamidine
Ocular effects	Cidofovir, ethambutol, rifabutin
Pancreatitis	Pentamidine, TMP-SMX, didanosine
Peripheral neuropathy	INH, ddI
Skin rash	Atovaquone, dapsone, sulfadiazine, TMP-SMX

NRTIs, NNRTIs, and Protease Inhibitors Licenced in the US for Treatment of HIV:

NUCLEOSIDE REVERSE TRANSCRIPTASE INHIBTORS (NRTI)	
Drug	**Common Adverse Effects**
Zidovidine (**AZT**) (Retrovir)	Anemia
Didanosine (**ddI**) (Videx)	GI upset, pancreatitis
Zalcitabine (**ddC**) (Hivid)	Neuropathy
Stavudine (**d4T**) (Zerit)	Neuropathy
Lamivudine (**3TC**) (Epivir)	Rare
Abacavir (**ABC**) (Ziagen)	Rash, fever
Non-Nucleoside Reverse Transcriptase Inhibtors (NNRTI)	
Nevirapine (Viramune)	Rash
Delavirdine (Rescriptor)	Rash
Efavirenz (Sustiva)	Altered mental status
PROTEASE INHIBITORS	
Ritonavir (Norvir)	GI upset, paresthesias
Indinavir (Crixivan)	Nephrolithiasis
Saquinavir (Fortovase)	Nausea
Nelfinavir (Viracept)	Diarrhea
Amprenavir (Agenerase)	Nausea

DDX OF NIGHT SWEATS
1. Pulmonary TB
2. Lymphoma
3. Brucellosis; abscess; endocarditis
4. Alcoholic withdrawal
5. Nocturnal hypoglycemia
6. Nocturnal dyspnea
7. Nightmares

FUO (FEVER OF UNKNOWN ORIGIN)—A GALLIUM SCAN WILL AID IN LOCALIZING THE FOLLOWING:
1. Abscess
2. Hepatoma
3. Lymphoma
4. Sarcoidosis

REMEMBER, AMONG THE MOST COMMON CAUSES OF FUO ARE:
1. Malignancy
2. TB
3. Abscess

DIRECT MICROSCOPY IN INFECTIOUS DISEASE

1. Acid-fast bacteria to Ziehl-Neelsen staining→mycobacteria species
2. Weakly acid-fast organisms
   a. Nocardia (aerobic)
   b. Actinomyces Israelii(anaerobic)
3. Dark-field examination→Treponema pallidum
4. Silver Methenamine stain→Pneumocystis carinii
5. India ink stain (CSF)→Cryptococcus neoformans
6. Gram-negative diplococci within leukocytes (endocervical/urethral swab)→N. gonorrhea
7. Inclusion bodies within urethral epithelial cells→Chlamydia trachomatis
8. Pyogenic meningitis in adults:

CSF gram stain	Presumptive diagnosis
Gram +	Strep pneumonia meningitis
Gram -	Meningococcal meningitis

THE BACTERIA

PSEUDOMONAS AERUGINOSA
1. Common organism leading to **infections complicating burns**
2. Cause of **malignant otitis externa in diabetics**
3. May cause **ecthyma gangrenosum in neutropenic patients** with bacteremia

SALMONELLA TYPHI→TYPHOID FEVER
1. Fever
2. Relative bradycardia
3. Rose spots (50% of pts)

BORDETELLA PERTUSSIS
1. Responsible for whooping cough
2. Should R/O in cases of prolonged bronchitis in older children and adults
3. May cause ↑↑Lymphocytes
4. Treatment with Erythromycin

CHLAMYDIA PSITTACOSIS
1. Asymptomatic avian carriers→poultry workers, e.g. cleaning out bird cages
2. F/C, H/A, dry cough, stiff neck; TCN is treatment.

LEGIONNAIRES'S DISEASE

1. Clinical: weakness, malaise, **high fever**, **cough**, and **diarrhea**, relative bradycardia, **bilateral** **patchy infiltrates**
2. Labs: **↓Na, ↓ Phos**, ↑ WBC, **↑ LFTs**
3. **Diagnosis: √ Ab with IFA (Indirect fluorescent Ab) test; ≥ 1:256 or a 4-fold ↑ is pos.**
4. Treatment: Erythro ± Rifampin; Fluoroquinolone; or Azithromax

PASTEURELLA MULTOCIDA

1. *Cat* (>dog)modes is the #1 mode of transmission
2. Pen G best, but Amox or Augmentin fine

CAPNOCYTOPHAGIA (aka 'DF-2')

1. *Dog* (> > cat) bites
2. Give Augmentin or Clindamycin
3. May cause bacteremia in immunosuppressed patients, splenectomized patients, and alcoholics.

COMPARISON:	**CAT SCRATCH DISEASE**	vs.	**BACILLARY ANGIOMATOSIS**
	Immunocompetent host		*Immunosuppressed* host(e.g. AIDS)
	Bartonella henselae (and A. felis)		Bartonella henselae (and quintana)
	Self-limited		*Progressive/recurrent*
	(spontaneous resolution in 2-4mo)		*Erythro or Doxy ±prophylaxis*

LISTERIA MONOCYTOGENES

1. Small, gram +, motile rod;
2. Causes aseptic meningitis/bacteremia in neonates, *immunosuppressed (e.g. lymphoma) and pregnant women*;
3. Associated with consumption of contaminated milk, ice cream, undercooked hot dogs
4. Rx→Amp + Gent

CLOSTRIDIUM BOTULINUM ('BOTULISM')

- Neurotoxin interferes with presynaptic Ach release, causing the 6D's→Dilated fixed pupils; Diplopia; Dysarthria; Dysphagia; Dry tongue; Descending paralysis.

NEISSERIA GONORRHEA

1. Gram negative diplococci
2. Look out for the 20 y.o. man or woman with **fever + swollen knee**
3. >80% of women are asymptomatic; only 2% of men asymptomatic.
4. Disseminated gonorrhea most likely to occur in menstruating females; 2 phases...
   a) **Bacteremic phase**: tenosynovitis; skin lesions; joint cultures negative
   b) **Nonbacteremic phase**:monoarticular arthritis of knee/wrist/ankle; joint cx pos

5. Remember, if a patient has a history of **recurrent** Neisseria infections, s/he probably has a deficiency in late complement components (C5-8). This is **best screened for with CH50**
6. Patients with GC should also be empirically treated for Chlamydia because of the high risk of co-occurrence. This can be accomplished with any number of available regimens (see "Treatment of STDs" later in this chapter for details)

NEISSERIA MENINGITIS
1. Gram negative diplococci
2. Presentation: **fever, ↓BP, DIC, palpable purpura (purpura fulminans)**
3. **Treatment→PenG;** *Don't wait for cultures if you suspect!*
4. **Prophylaxis** for exposure (close contact): Options→

    a) **Cipro 500mg PO once**
    b) **Rifampin 600mg q12h x 4 doses**
    c) **Ceftriaxone 250mg IM x 1**

BRUCELLOSIS

Persons at risk—
1. Farmers; dairymen; livestock handlers; meat packers
2. Veterinary surgeons
3. Those who ingest unpasteurized dairy products, mostly, however, from sheep/goats in Italy/Greece/France/Mexico.

Presentation—
1. Fever, chills
2. Headache
3. Back pain
4. Arthralgias
5. Orchitis
6. Cough
7. Hepatomegaly/Splenomegaly
8. Endocarditis

Diagnosis
1. Blood Cultures
2. Bone Marrow Culture
3. Serology

Treatment
♦ Doxycycline + *either* Gent/Streptomycin

MYCOPLASMA PNEUMONIAE ('Walking Pneumonia')

1. Community-acquired pneumonia, esp in **young** patients
2. Cold agglutinin production ± **hemolytic anemia**
3. **Erythema Multiforme**, **Stevens-Johnson** Syndrome
4. Non-specific musculoskeletal and/or GI upset
5. Neurological effects—**Guillain-Barre**, cranial nerve palsies, polio-like syndrome, **aseptic meningitis**.
6. **Mononeuritis Multiplex**
7. **Erythromycin** is the drug of choice in the young patient with fever/dry cough/patchy bilateral **interstitial** infiltrates, and relatively benign exam. Don't give PCN.

DIPTHERIA

1. Toxin-mediated complications include…
   a) Myocarditis→CHF and dysrhythmias
   b) Polyneuritis
2. Respiratory muscles may be paralyzed
3. Diagnosis established by culture or fluorescent Ab staining of pharyngeal swab specimen
4. Isolate the patient and treat with antitoxin
5. While Erythromycin or PenG do not alter the course of disease, they do prevent transmission to susceptible hosts. Close contacts should be evaluated and treated with Abx if culture results are +, and Td toxoid should be given.

ACTINOMYCES ISRAELII

1. Anaerobic, gram +, branching, filamentous
2. Sulfur granules, or clumps of filaments, seen on pathology
3. May present with
   a) **Paramandibular infection with a chronic draining sinus usually preceded by** dental extraction
   b) **Chest wound infection**
   c) **Pulmonary abscess**
   d) **Rib destruction**
4. Can cause brain abscess more rarely
5. Check anaerobic culture for diagnosis

NOCARDIA

1. Aerobic, gram +, branching, filamentous
2. An opportunistic infection (usually occurring in immunosuppressed)
3. Presents as chronic pneumonitis and lung abscess
4. In patients with chronic pneumonia who develop neurologic symptoms→r/o Nocardia brain abscess.

RICKETTSIAL INFECTIONS

1. All these infections have an **insect vector**, *except for* Q fever

2. They all yield a **rash**, *except for* Q fever and Erlichiosis (below).

3. **Rocky Mt. Spotted Fever (RMSF)**→Erythematous and hemorrhagic macules and papules ***begin peripherally*** (wrists/forearms, ankles) ***and spread centripetally*** (to arms, thighs, trunk, face). Fever, H/A, myalgia common symptoms. Rash usually begins on the 4th day of the fever. ↓Na+ is seen in half the cases. RMSF is ***not seen in the Rocky Mt. States*** (Go figure!), but is most common in the **mid-Atlantic states (i.e. MD, VA, NC, and Geogia)**; transmitted by the American **dog tick**, Dermacentor variabilis. History of tick bite given in >80% of cases. Doxycycline 100 IV or PO BID x 7days.

4. **Q fever** may develop hepatitis and pneumonitis and is seen in meat packers

5. **Erlichiosis**

   a) **S**pring and **S**ummer, more common
   b) 'Spotless RMSF' (no rash), with fever, H/A, malaise, relative bradycardia
   c) ↓WBC, ↓platelets, ↑LFTs
   d) Self-limited, usually, yet treated with TCN since deaths have been reported
   e) Sometimes see morulae (Latin for "mulberry": the appearance of the cytoplasmic inclusion, a vacuolar cluster of Giemsa-stained ehrlichiae in phagocytes) are frequently seen in the *granulocytic* type (as opposed to monocytic type)

OSTEOMYELITIS

1. Staph aureus is the #1 cause of acute hematogenous osteomyelitis and the #1 organism in chronic osteomyelitis; suspect salmonella of course in sickle cell disease.
2. Vertebral osteomyelitis
   a) Staph aureus and Gram neg bacilli
   b) MRI best imaging modality since may also show adjacent epidural abscess

BACTERIAL MENINGITIS→EMPIRIC TREATMENT (Based on initial gram stain)…

CSF Gram Stain	**Most likely organism**	**Empiric Treatment**
Gram + cocci	Strep Pneumonia	Vanco + Ceftriaxone ± dexamethasone
Gram-neg cocci	N. Meningitidis	Pen G
Gram + bacilli	Listeria Monocytogenes	Amp + Gent
Gram - bacilli	H. flu, coliforms, Pseudomonas	Ceftazidime + Gent

SYPHILIS

SENSITIVITY OF VDRL IN 1°, 2°, LATENT, AND 3° SYPHILIS:

1. 1° syphilis→ Positive in 80%; reliably negative within 2 years of successful treatment
2. 2° syphilis→ Positive in 99%
3. Latent syphilis→Positive in 70% (may remain + for long periods despite successful tx)
4. Neurosyphilis→CSF positive in 50% (i.e. 50% false negative rate)

CHOOSING THE MOST APPROPRIATE TEST IN SUSPECTED SYPHILIS

- **1° (recent) exposure**
    1. Darkfield exam of the 1° chancre
    2. FTA-ABS is the first test to become positive

- **2° Syphilis**
    1. Darkfield exam if skin/mucosal lesions present
    2. VDRL

- **Screening** (pregnant women, prostitutes, contacts of cases)
    1. VDRL
    2. If positive→check FTA-ABS

- **Follow-up after therapy**
    1. VDRL at 3,6,12 months
    2. If titre hasn't ↓d after 12 mo→retreat

- **Exclusion of Neurosyphilis**
    - CSF FTA-ABS (rules out if negative)

DIAGNOSTIC SIGNIFICANCE OF SYPHILIS SEROLOGY

	FTA-ABS +	FTA-ABS -
VDRL +	Syphilis	False Positives
VDRL -	Early, Latent, Late, or Treated Syphilis; False -	True Negatives

TREATMENT OF SYPHILIS DEPENDS ON THE STAGE AND IS SURPRISINGLY SIMPLE:

1° (painless chancre)→**Benzathine** PCN G 2.4 Million Units IM **x 1**

2° (maculopapular rash; condyloma lata; F/malaise/hepatitis/mucosal patches or erosions
in mouth→ **Benzathine** PCN G 2.4 Million Units IM **x 1**

Latent (defined as positive serology but no clinical disease)
> **Early** (<1y)→ **Benzathine** PCN G 2.4 Million Units IM **x 1**

> **Late** (>1y or situation in which 1° infection was unrecognzied)→
> **Benzathine** PCN G 2.4 Million Units IM **weekly x 3**

3°/Neurosyphilis (may be either asymp plus a positive CSF VDRL *OR* symptomatic)→
PCN G 2-4M units **IV q4h x 10-14 days**→FOLLOWED BY…
Benzathine PCN G 2.4 Million Units IM **weekly x 3**

- *Follow sequential serum and CSF VDRL titres.*

IMPORTANT GRAM-STAINS:
1. **Gram + cocci**
   a. Staph
   b. Strep

2. **Gram - cocci (Neisseria species)**
   a. NM
   b. NG
   c. Moraxella Catarrhalis (aka Branhamella Catarralis)

3. **Gram + bacilli**
   a. Clostridium
   b. Bacillus species (e.g. B. cereus; B fragilis)
   c. Corynebacterium
   d. Actinomyces israeli
   e. Gardnerella vaginalis
   f. Listeria monocytogenes

4. **Gram - bacilli**
   a. Enterobacteriaceae (E. Coli, Proteus, Klebsiella, Salmonella, Shigella)
   b. Pseudomonas aeruginosa
   c. H. flu (actually a 'coccobacillus')
   d. Campylobacter jejuni
   e. Brucella

5. **Acid-fast bacilli (AFB)**
   a. Mycobacteria
   b. Nocardia asteroides (weakly acid-fast)

STREPTOCOCCAL INFECTIONS

3 MAIN CLINICAL GROUPS OF STREPTOCOCCI

1. **Strep Pyogenes ("Beta-hemolytic" Strep)**

    a) Acute invasive suppurative effects
       (1) **Impetigo**
       (2) **Cellulitis**
       (3) **Pharyngitis**

    b) Other acute sequelae
       (1) **Scarlet fever**
       (2) **Erysipelas**

    c) Late non-suppurative sequelae
       (1) **Rheumatic fever**
       (2) **Poststreptococcal glomerulonephritis**

2. **Strep Pneumoniae**

    a) Pneumonia (esp. community-acquired lobar)
    b) Otitis
    c) Meningitis

3. **Strep Viridans**—a broad term that includes (among others)

    a) **S. Faecalis** (enterococci)
       (1) UTI
       (2) Infective endocarditis (notoriously PCN-resistant)

    b) **S. Bovis** (enterococci)
       (1) Infective endocarditis (exquisitely PCN-sensitive)
       (2) remember, if + BC in infective endocarditis→√ colonoscopy for ca

CHARACTERIZATION OF STREPTOCOCCI

A. Classification by **Lancefield Ag groups:**
    a) *Group A Strep (Pyogenes)*
    b) *Group D Strep, e.g. Strep Bovis*→endocarditis→Treatment is PenG or Ceftriaxone, OR (if intermed sensitivity to PCN)→PenG + Gent
    c) *Enterococcus*--PCN is bacteriastatic, not bacteriacidal; resistant to all cephalosporins
       (1) E. faecalis→PCN G; add Gent for endocarditis or meningitis
       (2) E. faecium→No Abx regimen proven efficacious; multi-drug resistant (PCN, Aminoglycosides, and Vanco)

B.   Classification by in vitro **Hemolysis:**

   a)   *α-hemolytic:*

> (1)   **Strep Viridans→#1 cause of** non-IVDA **native valve endocarditis (Staph aureus #1 if IVDA and usually affects the tricuspid valve)**→Treatment same as for Strep Bovis

   (2)   Pneumococci

   b)   *β-hemolytic:* =Strep Pyogenes

   ◆   N.B. Strep Pyogenes and Pneumococcus rarely cause endocarditis

CLINICAL CORRELATIONS OF STREPTOCOCCAL INFECTIONS

1.   Untreated Group A Strep pharyngitis predisposes to development of rheumatic fever
2.   Remember, Strep A throat *and skin* infections→post-strep glomerulonephritis
3.   Prompt antibiotic therapy does not appear to prevent the development of post-strep glomerulonephritis, as compared to rheumatic fever following throat infection.

RHEUMATIC FEVER

1.   Acute Rheumatic Fever occurs only after **Group A Strep pharyngitis**, and never after Strep skin infections.

2.   Preventable by antibiotic therapy (PCN best) **within 7 days of onset of strep throat**. Monthly IM PCN or daily PO PCN or Erythromycin are used.

3.   Due to **cross-reactive anti-heart Abs stimulated by Group A strep**

4.   Major and Minor Jones Criteria: **"S.A.F.E.R. C.A.S.E.S."** ...
      (must have 2 major or 1major + 2 minor criteria to make the dx)

Minor	**Major**
Sore throat	**C**arditis
Arthralgias	**A**SO titre↑
Fever	**S**yndenham's chorea
EKG changes;↑ **E**SR	**E**rythema Marginatum
Rheumatic History	**S**Q nodules

5. **Rheumatic fever** is generally considered to be **an inflammatory disorder of connective tissue—an autoimmune response to untreated Group A β-Hemolytic Strep (GABHS) pharyngitis in a genetically predisposed host.**

6. *__Clinical manifestations usually appear 1-3 weeks after the onset of pharyngitis__.*

7. Although this self-limited, multisystem disease can affect heart, joints, brain, and cutaneous, and SQ tissues, **cardiac damage** *__is the only potentially chronic debilitating effect__. Carditis occurs in about 50%* of cases. Endocardial involvement with auscultatory evidence of MR or AI is required for diagnosis. Mild MR occurring as the sole cardiac manifestation during the acute attack will often disappear. AI occurring during the attack leads to permanent damage in 90% of patients.

8. *Migratory polyarthritis occurs in about 70%* of patients, characteristically shows rapid relief with ASA (usually within 48h) and *never* causes *permanent* joint damage.

9. **Treatment** is with an IM injection 1.2 M units benzathine Pen G.

10. ASA remains the anti-inflammatory of choice and should be started as soon as the diagnosis is suspected.

11. *__Rheumatic fever may recur with subsequent GABHS infections__.* Such recurrences can be prevented by appropriate **secondary prophylaxis** → PCN IM or PO (*or* Sulfadiazene or Eythromycin if pen-allergic)

MANAGEMENT OF ACUTE RHEUMATIC FEVER:

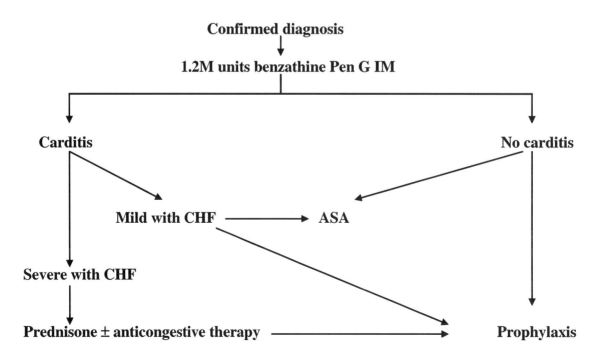

DURATION OF <u>SECONDARY PROPHYLAXIS</u>:	
Patient Type	**Duration**
Rheumatic fever with carditis and residual heart disease	≥10y since last episode and ≥ until 40 yo, whichever is longer; some recommend lifelong prophylaxis
Rheumatic fever with carditis but no residual heart disease	10y or well into adulthood whichever is longer
Rheumatic fever without carditis	5y or until 21yo, whichever is longer

IMPORTANT INDICATIONS FOR VANCOMYCIN

1. Bacterial endocarditis—PCN allergy and prosthetic valve involvement
2. Enterococcus faecalis
3. MRSA
4. PCN-Resistant Strep Pneumoniae
5. Pseudomembranous colitis

IMPORTANT INDICATIONS FOR METRONIDAZOLE

1. Abscesses
2. Amebiasis
3. Anaerobic infections
4. Gardnerella vaginitis (Bacterial vaginosis)
5. Giardiasis
6. Trichomoniasis

CLASSIFICATION OF QUINOLONE ANTIBIOTICS:		
Classification	**Agent**	**Antimicrobial spectrum**
First generation	Nalidixic acid (NegGram®) Cinoxacin (Cinobac®)	Gram-negatives (but no Pseudomonas)
Second generation	Norfloxacin (Noroxin®) Lomefloxacin (Maxaquin®) Enoxacin (Penetrex®) Ofloxacin (Floxin®) Ciprofloxacin (Cipro®)	Gram-negatives (including Pseudomonas), some gram + (Staph aureus but not Strep pneumoniae) and some atypicals
Third generation	Levofloxacin (Levaquin®) Sparfloxacin (Zagam®) Gatifloxacin (Tequin®) Moxifloxacin (Avelox®)	Same as for 2nd gen plus expanded gram + coverage (Pen-sensitive and Pen-resistant Strep pneumoniae) + expanded activity vs. atypicals
Fourth generation	Trovafloxacin (Trovan®)	Same as for 3rd gen + broad anaerobic coverage

TETANUS PROPHYLAXIS IN WOUND MANAGEMENT (30th ed. Sanford Guide)

History of Tetanus Immunization	Clean Minor Wounds		Dirty, Tetanus-prone Wound	
	TD[12]	TIG	Td	TIG
Unknown or < 3doses*	Yes	*No*	Yes	Yes
≥3 doses**	No[3]	No	No[4]	No

* *"YES" to all except clean TIG !*
** *"NO" to all !*

MECHANISMS OF VACCINE ACTION
1. **Toxoids:**
    a) Tetanus
    b) Diptheria
    c) Botulism

2. **Recombinant vaccines:**
    a) Hep B
    b) Cholera

3. **Pooled surface proteins:**
    a) Strep Pneumococcus
    b) H. Flu B (HiB)

4. **Attenuated (live) organisms**, **CONTRAINDICATED in PREGNANT OR IMMUNOCOMPROMISED pts!**
    a) Polio
    b) M, M, and R (all three)
    c) BCG
    d) Yellow fever
    e) Rabies
    f) VZV (Varicella-Zoster)

5. **Killed organisms***:*
    a) Influenza B
    b) Hep A
    c) Typhoid
    d) Pertussis

---

[1]   Td=Tetanus & diptheria toxoids adsorbed (adults)
    TIG=Tetanus Immune Globulin
[2]   Yes if wound > 24 hours old
    For children < 7yo, DPT (DT if pertussis vaccine contraindicated)
    For persons ≥ 7 yo, Td preferred to tetanus toxoid alone

[3]   Yes if over 5 years since last booster
[4]   Yes if over 10 years since last booster

ENDOCARDITIS ANTIBIOTIC PROPHYLAXIS In Patients With Underlying Heart Disease:

Prophylaxis Recommended	Prophylaxis *NOT* Recommended
Cardiac conditions	Negligible Risk
High risk	ASD (*secundum*;=right axis deviation)
Prosthetic valves	MVP without MR
Prev bacterial endocarditis	Physiologic/functional/
Cyanotic congenital heart disease	or innocent heart
Moderate risk	murmurs
IHSS	Pacemakers
MVP with regurgitation, or	IADs (implantable automatic
thickening of MV leaflets	defibrillators)
Dental	
Extractions	
Periodontal procedures	Routine cavity filling with local anesthesthetic
Respiratory	
Rigid Bronchoscopy	Flexible bronchoscopy
Tonsillectomy/Adenoidectomy	
GI	
Sclerotherapy of esoph varices	TEE
Dilatation of esoph stricture	EGD without biopsy
ERCP with biliary tract obstruction	
Biliary tract surgery	
GU	
Prostate surg; cystoscopy	Vag hysterectomy/delivery; C sx

> ***IMPORTANT RULES OF THUMB***:
> - Most congenital heart disease (**except secundum ASD**) requires procedural antibiotic prophylaxis.
> - **MVP with incompetence/murmur** needs antibiotic prophylaxis.

OCCURRENCE OF INFECTIVE ENDOCARDITIS (In ↓ing Order)

1. Primary (40%)→**Strep Viridans**

2. Previous Rheumatic Valve Damage (30%)→Strep Viridans

3. Congenital Heart disease (10%)

4. **Prosthetic valve** (10%)→**Staph Epidermidis**

5. IVDA (10%)→Staph Aureus; Tricuspid valve

6. **Colon Ca→Strep Bovis**

TREATMENT

1. **Native valve endocarditis**
   a) Strep Viridans→Pen G ± Gent
   b) Enterococci→Treatment depends on resistance to PCN/Aminoglycs/Vanco
   c) MSSA→Nafcillen (or oxacillen) + Gent
   d) MRSA→Vancomycin
   e) HACEK organisms (fastidious, slow-growing, Gram neg bacilli)→Ceftriaxone
   f) Culture negative→Treatment depends on the specific causal organism (i.e. Q fever, bartonella, brucellosis, psittacosis, or fungi)

2. *Empiric* **therapy (culture pending) for NATIVE VALVE endocarditis**→ (PCN *or* Amp *or* Naf *or* Ox) + Gent; Vanco & Gent if Pen-allergic.

3. *Empiric* **therapy for PROSTHETIC VALVE** endocarditis→Vanco + Gent + Rifampin

4. **Culture positive prosthetic valve** infection→Surgical consult *PLUS*
   a) Staph epidermidis (usually a contaminant on BC) →Vanco + Gent + Rifampin
   b) MSSA→Nafcillen + Gent
   c) MRSA→ Vanco + Gent
   d) Strep Viridans→same as for native valve above
   e) Candida or Aspergillus→Ampho B ± Fluconazole

INDICATIONS FOR SURGERY IN INFECTIVE ENDOCARDITIS
1. Massive vegetations seen on echo
2. Persistent bacteremias/fevers despite optimal medical mgmt
3. Prosthetic valve involvement
4. Refractory CHF, esp with AI
5. Repeated septic emboli
6. Suspected extensive valve ring infection
7. Hemolysis
8. Conduction disturbances (associated with abscess)

POST-SPLENECTOMY INFECTIONS

Clearly involved
1. Strep Pneumoniae
2. DF-2 bacillus
3. Malaria
4. Babesiosis

Probably involved
1. H. Flu
2. Neisseria Meningitidis

Possibly involved
1. Beta-hemolytic Strep
2. E. Coli
3. Pseudomonas
4. Staph Aureus

TREATMENT OF STDs (PER SANFORD GUIDE AND CDC)

STD	Treatment Guidelines
Chancroid	Azithromycin single dose of 1g PO; or Ceftriaxone 250mg IM x1; or Erythro 500 qid x 1 week
Chlamydia trachomatis	Azithromycin single dose of 1g PO; or Doxy 100 BID x 1 week
GC, uncomplicated	Cipro 500 PO x1 or Ofloxacin 400 PO x1 or Ceftriaxone 125 IM x 1 or Cefixime 400 PO x 1
HSV, genital, primary	Acyclovir 400 TID x 10d; or Famvir 250 TID x 5-10d; or Valtrex 1000 BID x 10d
Lymphogranuloma Venereum (LGV)	Doxycycline 100 BID x 3 weeks
Syphilis	See section on Syphilis, since treatment depends on stage of disease.
Trichomonas vaginalis ('Trich')	Metronidazole 2g PO x 1; contraindicated in 1st trimester preg

VAGINITIS—3 MAIN TYPES:

VAGINITIS	CLINICAL FINDINGS	TREATMENT
Candida albicans	**'Cottage cheese curds'; no odor; pruritic; common after Abx and in obese or diabetics.**	**Fluconazole 150 PO x1; or intravaginal azole**
Trichomoniasis	**Yellow, purulent discharge; 'Strawberry cervix' seen on culposcopy 2° petechia seen; Dx usu. by wet mount**	**Metronidazole 2g PO x 1;** *contraindicated in 1st trimester pregnancy; must also treat sexual partner*
Gardnerella vaginalis ('Bacterial Vaginosis')	**Malodorous "fishy" smell after adding KOH ('whiff test'); 'clue cells' on wet mount.**	**Metronidazole 2g PO x 1** *less effective than* **PO or intravaginal dosing x 5-7 days**

EPIDIDYMITIS: THE *RULE OF THUMB*:
⇒ Men <35=Chlamydia or GC→ Treat as for **GC + Chlamydia** (see STD table above)
⇒ Men >35=**E. Coli** usually→Treat with TMP-SMX or Ciprofloxacin.

DERMATOLOGIC INFECTIONS COMMON IN AIDS:

1. **Herpes Zoster** (shingles)→VZV

2. **Oral hairy leukoplakia** →EBV and usually seen in advanced AIDS. Treatment is acyclovir / antivirals (*Note*: this is **_not_ the same as "oral leukoplakia"**, which is related to HPV, smoking, smokeless tobacco, alcohol, and syphilis. Candida can invade oral leukoplakia secondarily, and it is considered a premalignant lesion for squamous cell ca)

3. **Molluscum contagiosum**→Discrete, solid, skin-colored papules that are only 1-2 mm in diameter, have **central umbilication**

4. **Bacillary angiomatosis** (vascular papules or nodules caused by **Bartonella** (Rochalimaea) henselae and quintana and transmitted by cats or ticks)→Erythromycins or Doxycycline for treatment

LABORATORY CHARACTERIZATION OF GENITAL ULCERS

1. **Positive dark-field exam**→1° syphilis

2. *H. Ducreyi* on microscopy→**Chancroid**

3. **Donovan bodies** on microscopy→**Granuloma inguinale (Donovanosis); caused by...** *Calymmatobacterium granulomatis* [1° Rx=Doxy or Bactrim x 3 weeks; alt Rx=Ery or Cipro also x 3 weeks]

4. *Chlamydia* on culture/serology→**LGV** (Lymphogranuloma venereum)

5. Herpes simplex on viral cultures

6. **Negative microbiology→consider Behcet's/Reiter's** syndrome

AMINOGLYCOSIDE TOXICITY

• The **nephrotoxicity is almost always reversible;** NSAIDs, Vanco, Ampho enhance

• The **ototoxicity** is almost always *IR*reversible; loop diuretics enhance

• **Mg, K+, Ca : wasting**

FUNGAL INFECTIONS

COCCIDIOIDES IMMITIS
1. **San Joaquin Valley, California**
2. **Central Arizona**
3. Dissemination most likely to occur in males, esp Filipino and blacks
4. Primary infection is pneumonitis; see dry cough, fever, and pleural effusion
5. E. Nodosum may be seen
6. Hilar adenopathy common
7. Diagnosis by complement fixation (titre $\geq$ 1:4)
8. PO Fluconazole (Diflucan®) is the treatment

HISTOPLASMOSIS
1. **Ohio and Mississippi River valleys**
2. Associated with cleaning chicken coops/bird nesting areas→exposure to **bird droppings**.
3. Patients are usually **immunocompetent**
4. Colonic involvement in AIDS
5. 2 forms:
    a) Primary (acute) form→resembles flu/URI
    b) Chronic cavity disease→Bilateral upper lung distribution, similar to TB
6. Itraconazole, Ampho B are the treatment options depending on severity/immune status.

BLASTOMYCOSIS
1. Affects lungs, skin, bone, and prostate/epididymis/testes
2. **Cutaneous** is most common clinical form
3. Itraconazole or Ampho B depending on severity

- **The major advantage of Itraconazole over Fluconazole is its greater activity against Aspergillus, Sporothrix, Histoplasmosis, and Blastomycosis.**

ASPERGILLOSIS THE FOUR PATTERNS OF PULMONARY INFECTION
1. Saprophytic infections (2° infection in necrotic tissue)
2. **Chronic Necrotizing Aspergillosis**→ especially in *preexisting pulmonary bullous disease*—e.g. TB or ankylosing spondylitis)→look for **ASPERGILLOMA** (fungal ball)
    a) Anti-fungal therapy not helpful
    b) Surgery for patients with hemoptysis
3. **ABPA (Allergic Bronchopulmonary Aspergillosis)**
    a) Presents as **asthma** with wheezing and brown mucus plugs
    b) Commonly seen in asthmatics who have been stable on chronic maintenance therapy and suddenly *breaks through*.

      c) *Diagnosis*
         i)   Clinical presentation
           (a) May cause sinus and pulmonary infection in neutropenic patients
           (b) **Migratory pulmonary infiltrates**
           (c) Presentation of chronic granulomatous disease in a young patient may be an Aspergillus infection.
        ii) Aspergillus precipitans in blood
        iii) Wheal-and-flare (immediate Type 1) skin test reactivity
        iv) ↑ Total IgG in blood
        v) ↑ **Total IgE** and Aspergillus-specific Ab
        vi) **Peripheral blood ↑eos**
        vii) + Sputum culture for Aspergillus (beware, though, since it is a frequent colonizer)

      ❂ **TREATMENT IS STEROIDS.**
      ❂ **THERE IS NO ROLE FOR ANTIFUNGALTHERAPY IN ABPA.**

4. **Invasive Bronchopulmonary Disease**
      a) Prolonged neutropenia predisposes, especially in
         i)   AML
         ii) CLL
         iii) Hodgkin's
      b) Ampho B or itraconazole

CRYPTOCOCCUS NEOFORMANS
1. Most infections occur in **immunosuppressed** patients (as opposed to Histo)

2. *Similar* to Histo, however, **pigeon droppings** may play a role

3. **Meningitis** is most common form of infection, and if C. Neoformans is isolated from anywhere→must √ the CSF

4. Treatment
      a) Non-meningeal, Non-AIDS→Ampho til response, then Fluconazole; or Fluconazole alone
      b) *Meningitis*, Non-AIDS→Ampho B + Flucytosine til afebrile & culture neg, →then PO Fluconazole; or Fluconazole alone
      c) HIV+/AIDS (usually *meningitis*)→Ampho B + Flucytosine→then PO Fluconazole indefinitely

CANDIDA
1. Immunosuppressed + infected intravenous catheters→Candidemia
2. IVDA→can see Candida albicans (and other Candida species) endocarditis
3. Hepatic candidiasis seen commonly in neutropenic patients following bone marrow transplant.
4. Causes oral & esophageal candidiasis in immunosuppressed
5. Ampho B/Fluconazole

SPOROTRICHOSIS

1. An ulceronodular dermatosis caused by Sporothrix schenckii, a fungus commonly found in *soil, and usually affecting gardeners*, farmers, florists, lawn workers. Chronic nodular lymphagitis and regional lymphadenitis are concomitant
2. Pulmonary infection may lead to empyema, chronic pneumonitis, cavities

MUCOR

1. Caused by Rhizopus, Zygomycetes
2. *DKA* or immunosuppressed + Mucormycosis→rhinocerebral infections
3. Diagnosis based on finding **black, necrotic lesions** around the eyes, nose, soft/hard palates;
4. Biopsy confirmatory.
5. *Ampho B + surgical debridement*

PARASITIC INFECTIONS

GIARDIA.

1. Recognize it as a potential pathogen in **white water rafting trips**; be able to recognize it's microscopic appearance.
2. Clinical: sudden onset of **watery diarrhea, bloating, flatulence**
3. The treatment is **metronidazole**.

AMEBIASIS

1. **AMEBIC LIVER ABSCESS**
   a) *Right* lobe effected in 90% of cases
   b) *Males* affected in 80% of cases
   c) *Single* abscess seen in 70% of cases; the fluid on aspiration has been said to resemble "chocolate syrup" or "anchovy paste".
   d) *Normal LFTs*, usually.

   - You can *remember these* by recalling, "**Ame is looking for a normal, single, male, Mr. Right**"!

   e) Stools may contain cysts and may be difficult to distinguish from leukocytes.
   f) Patients with hepatic abscess usually don't have the diarrhea
2. **Bloody diarrhea**
3. Serology, using complement fixation testing is positive in >90%

TOXOPLASMOSIS

1. Acquired from eating undercooked meat or exposure to **cat** feces
2. *Disorders in the normal host:*
   a) **Mono-like syndrome**
   b) **Ocular toxoplasmosis**
      i) Usually the result of congenital infections
      ii) Characteristic lesion is focal necrotizing retinitis tht initially appears in the fundus as yellowish-white, elevated, cotton patches with indistinct margins, usually on the posterior pole
      iii) Presents with blurred vision, scotoma, pain, photophobia
      iv) *Treatment: Pyrimethamine + Sulfadiazene + Leucovorin (folate); Steroids indicated if lesions involve the macula or optic nerve head*
   c) Congenital toxo (part of the TORCH syndrome)

3. *Disorders of the immunodeficient patient*
   a) Brain lesions (often difficult to ddx with CNS lymphoma, since both give ring-enhancing lesions)
   b) Myocarditis
   c) Pneumonia

MALARIA

1. Transmitted by the bite of the Anopheles mosquito
2. Plasmodium is the parasite and has 4 species
   a) P. *vivax*→Chloroquine + Primaquine
   b) P. *ovale*→Chloroquine + Primaquine
   c) P. *falciparum*→Chloroquine; if resistant to Chloroquine then→ PO Primaquine or Azithromax; if too ill for PO, then give IV Quinidine
   d) P. *malariae*→Chloroquine
3. **Presentation**
   a) High Fever→may see seizures
   b) Normochromic, normocytic anemia 2° to…
   c) Hemolysis→Hemoglobinuria→*blackish* urine
   d) Low BP/Shock/DIC
   e) Low glucose (poor prognosticator)
   f) Coma 2° to encephalopathy

4. Diagnosis made by examining **thick and thin smears**

5. **Prophylaxis…**
   a) **Chloroquine** is the first choice: 500mg PO q week, *starting 1-2 weeks prior to travel and stopping 4 weeks after return.*
   b) For Chlorquine-*resistant* areas→**Mefloquine** (*contraindicated* for patients on *Beta-blockers*)
   c) For Chloroquine & Mefloquine-resistant areas→Doxycycline
   d) Patient should be advised to take 3 tabs at once of pyrimethamine-sulfadoxine should fever develop in areas endemic for malaria.

7. DERMATOLOGY

✪ SKIN DISEASE AS A MANIFESTATION OF MALIGNANCY...

1. **Acanthosis nigricans** (not just DM and obesity!)→GI malignancy, esp gastric, ovarian.

2. **Actinic keratosis**→Squamous cell carcinoma

3. **Café au lait spots**→ Von Recklinghausen's disease

4. **Dysplastic nevus**→Malignant melanoma

5. **Epidermal cysts, fibromas, lipomas**→Gardner's syndrome;

6. **Flushing, telangiectasias**→Carcinoid tumors

7. **Mucosal hyperpigmentation** (esp. lips)→ Peutz-Jeghers syndrome

8. **Necrolytic erythematous rash**→Glucagonoma

9. **Erythroderma**→ Sezary syndrome (rare variant of cutaneous T-cell lymphoma, aka mycosis fungoides), mycosis fungoides

10. **Dermatomyositis** (esp. steroid-resistant form in adults)→Many types of cancers, esp ovarian/gastric/lung ca.; look for heliotrope rash/Gottron's papules/violaceous erythematous rash

11. **Post-proctoscopic periorbital 'pinch' purpura**→Myeloma with 2° amyloidosis

12. **Acquired ichthyosis**→Hodgkin's Disease

13. **Hirsutism**→PCO (Polycystic Ovary Syndrome); adrenal or ovarian tumors (2° to androgen excess)

14. **Erythema gyratum repens**→Classically associated with breast ca

15. **Sweet's syndrome** (acute febrile neutrophilic dermatosis)→AML; Sweet's syndrome is characterized by painful plaque-forming inflammatory papules and associated with Fever, arthralgias, and peripheral ↑WBC. Note, the fever/arthralgias/splenomegaly/ ↑WBC is similar to Still's Disease

16. **Generalized pruritis**→May be indicative of lymphoma

17. **Tylosis (palmar/plantar keratoderma)**→Esophageal carcinoma;

18. **Pemphigus**→Thymoma ± myasthenia gravis

19. **Bullous pemphigoid**→Has not been associated with any underlying malignancy

20. **Ashleef spots**→Tuberous sclerosis (also associated with mental retardation, seizures, and renal angiomyolipomas)

✪ CUTANEOUS SIGNS OF SYSTEMIC DISEASE...

1. **Pyoderma Gangrenosum**→IBD (UC> Crohn's); Rheumatoid Arthritis

2. **Heliotrope rash** (periorbital discoloration)→Dermatomyositis

3. **Lupus Pernio** (erythematous swelling of the nose) and Erythema Nodosum→sarcoidosis

4. E. Nodosum + Fever + arthralgias + bilateral hilar LN→=**Lofgren's Syndrome**, with which acute sarcoidosis may present;

5. **Pseudoxanthoma elasticum** (yellow xanthomatous papules seen on the abdomen/groin/neck/axilla→ ↑ risk of CVA, MI, PVD, MVP, angioid streaks in the retina

6. **Ehlers-Danlos syndrome** (skin hyperextensibility + joint hypermobility) →↑ risk of angina, PVD, MVP, GI bleed

7. Hereditary hemorrhagic telangiectasia (**Osler-Weber-Rendu**)=cutaneous and mucosal telangiectasias → associated with nosebleeds, GI bleeds, pulmonary AVMs, and CNS angiomas;

8. **Acrodermatitis enteropathics** →Zinc deficiency ± alopecia, diarrhea

9. **Dermatitis herpetiformis** (immune-mediated bullous disease)→Celiac disease (gluten-sensitive enteropathy)

10. **Apthous ulcers**→Celiac disease; Crohn's disease; Behcet's disease; Reiter's Syndrome; HIV

11. **Mucosal/Labial hyperpigmentation**→Peutz-Jeghers syndrome (no ↑ risk of developing ca)

12. **Erythema Chronicum Migrans**→Lyme Disease

13. **C.R.E.S.T.** (**variant of scleroderma**)=Calcinosis cutis; Raynaud's phenomenon; Esophageal dysmotility; Sclerodactyly; and Telangiectasias

14. **Livedo Reticularis**; this is a mottled bluish (livid) discoloration of the skin that looks like a net. It is not a diagnosis per se, but more a reaction pattern to vasculitis syndromes, drugs, atheroemboli.

15. **Morphea** (discrete sclerotic plaques with white shiny center)→Scleroderma

16. **Eosinophilic Fasciitis** (tightly bound thickening of skin and underlying tissues)→Scleroderma;

17. Erythematous macular-papular eruption of trunk/palms/soles after BMT→**GVHD**

18. **Necrobiosis lipoidica diabeticorum** (yellow-brown atrophic telangiectatic plaques on the shins)→Diabetes Mellitus

19. **Pretibial Myxedema** (pink- and skin-colored papules, plaques, and nodules, usually occurring on the shins)→Graves' disease. Do not confuse this dermatologic myxedema with the myxedema associated with Hypothyroidism ("Myxedema coma")

20. **Toxic Epidermal Necrolysis and Stevens-Johnson Syndrome**→mucocutaneous usually *drug-induced* skin tenderness and erythema, followed by extensive exfoliation

21. **Janeway lesions**→ Infective endocarditis. *Nontender*, hemorrhagic, infarcted macules and papules on the fingers, palms, soles; in contrast to **Osler's nodes**, which have a similar distribution and are seen in infective endocarditis, but are *tender.*

22. **SSSS (Staphylococcal Scalded-Skin Syndrome)**-A Staph aureus *toxin-mediated* painful, tender, diffuse erythema that is followed by desquamation and occurring mainly in newborns and infants under 2 yo

23. **Toxic Shock Syndrome**—Similar to SSSS, it is a Staph aureus *toxin-mediated* illness that causes Fever, Hypotension, generalized skin and mucosal erythema, and multisystem failure occurring in menstrual and nonmenstrual patterns

24. **"Salmon-colored"** rash + arthralgias + ↑ WBC + Fever + Splenomegaly→*Still's Disease.*

25. **Cushing's Syndrome**→ "buffalo hump" (fat pad), purple striae (usu. on the abdomen), hirsutism, steroid acne

CUTANEOUS MANIFESTATIONS IN INFECTIOUS DISEASE

1. **Keratoderma Blenorrhagicum** (vesicular rash on the palms/soles that crusts)→*Reiter's Syndrome* (other signs include conjunctivitis, uveitis, urethritis, and arthritis); rash known differently as **Circinate Ballinitis** if affects the glans penis

2. **Ampicillen (or Amoxicillin) + Infectious Mono (EBV or CMV)**→ Almost all patients develop a Morbilliform rash, defined as an exanthematous (viral-like) drug eruption, often mimicking rash of measles

3. **Measles**→A maculopapular rash that *spreads from the head down and resolves in the same order* after approximately 3 days

4. **Rocky Mt. Spotted Fever (RMSF)**→Erythematous and hemorrhagic macules and papules *begin peripherally* (wrists/forearms, ankles) *and spread centripetally* to arms, thighs, trunk, face. Fever, H/A, myalgia typically accompany

5. **Ecthyma Gangrenosum**→ A cellulitis with necrosis related to septic vasculitis. It begins with cutaneous infarction and progresses to large, ulcerated gangrenous lesions. The causative organism is *Pseudomonas Aeruginosa*; the patient is usually immunocompromised/neutropenic and bacteremia is common

6. **Impetigo**→*crusted golden-yellow erosions* which become confluent on the nose, cheeks, chin, and lips 2° to Staph Aureus and Group A Strep (Pyogenes)

7. **Erysipelas**→ Red, painful cellulitis 2° to Staph aureus, but more commonly group A Strep. The margins of the cellulitis are raised, and the borders are sharply demarcated

8. **Erysipeloid**→A violaceous erythematous cellulitis to the hand 2° to Erysipelothrix rhusiopathiae after handling saltwater fish, shellfish, meat, hides, poultry. (DDx is V. Vulnificus)

9. **Desquamation + Strawberry tongue**→*Scarlet fever* 2° to Group A Strep; Kawasaki disease may also give a Strawberry tongue + a Desquamating rash.

10. **Purpura Fulminans**→The cutaneous manifestation of DIC or *acute meningococcemia*; the less fulminant cases of meningococcemia may manifest as a more discrete petechial rash

11. **Cat Scratch Disease**→caused by *Bartonella henselae* (formerly Rochalimaea henselae) and is a *benign, self-limiting* infection characterized by a primary skin or conjunctival lesion, following cat scratches or contact with a cat, and subsequent tender regional lymphadenopathy. Unlike Bacillary angiomatosis, also caused by Bartonella, antibiotics have not proved effective in treatment

12. **Rosacea**—A chronic acneform disorder of the facial pilosebaceous units. ↑ capillary sensitivity to heat results in flushing and ultimately telangiectasia. Long-standing disease with edema and hyperplasia of the skin overlying the nose, cheeks, and forehead leads to *Rhinophyma*

13. **Pityriasis Versicolor**→A chronic, asymptomatic scaling rash caused by the *hyphal* form of Pityrosporum ovale, characterized by well-demarcated scaling patches with variable hyperpigmentation, usually occurring on the trunk. Diagnosis confirmed by a + KOH prep. *It's other name is Tinea Versicolor*. Treatment is antifungals, like ketoconazole or itraconazole or topical azole creams, selenium sulfide, or propylene glycol.

14. **Pityriasis Rosea**—Distinctive rash that *begins as a "herald patch"*, *usually on the trunk*, followed 1-2 weeks later with a generalized exanthematous eruption that resolves spontaneously after 6 weeks without therapy. More common in the *spring and fall.* May be 2° to picornavirus.

15. **Sporotrichosis**—An ulceronodular dermatosis caused by Sporothrix schenckii, a fungus commonly found in *soil, and usually affecting gardeners*, farmers, florists, lawn workers. Chronic nodular lymphagitis and regional lymphadenitis are concomitant

16. STD's (chancroid, chancre, etc)→see ID lecture. However, should remember that *among the genital ulcers,* Chancroid, HSV, and Behc et's→ *are PAINFUL;* Syphilis (Syphi<u>LESS</u>), LGV, and Granuloma Inguinale→ *are pain<u>LESS</u>*

DERMATOLOGY AND AIDS

1. **Kaposi's sarcoma**—oval papules or purplish plaques on the trunk, extremities, face, mucosa;

2. **Herpes Zoster** (shingles)→VZV

3. **Oral hairy leukoplakia** ✪ →EBV and usually seen in advanced AIDS. (This is *__not the same as__* "oral leukoplakia", which is related to HPV, smoking, smokeless tobacco, alcohol, and syphilis. Candida can invade oral leukoplakia secondarily, and it is considered a premalignant lesion for squamous cell ca)

4. **Molluscum contagiosum** ✪→Discrete, solid, skin-colored papules that are only 1-2 mm in diameter, have central umbilication

5. **Bacillary angiomatosis** ✪ (vascular papules or nodules caused by Bartonella (Rochalimaea) henselae and quintana and transmitted by cats or ticks)→Erythromycins or Doxycycline for rx.

2 TONGUE DISORDERS THAT LOOK HIGHLY ABNORMAL, BUT REQUIRE ONLY REASSURANCE...

1. **Fissured** tongue (aka scrotal tongue)
2. **Geographic** tongue (migratory glossitis)

GRANULOMA ANNULARE

1. Self-limiting, asymptomatic, chronic dermatosis commonly on the dorsa of the hands/feet/elbows/knees

2. A local dermatosis, and not indicative of systemic or underlying disease

3. Although asymptomatic and not indicative of systemic disease, it can be cosmetically disfiguring and treatment with application of steroids (local disease) or PUVA photochemotherapy (if generalized GA)

SQUAMOUS CELL CA

1. **RISK FACTORS** ✪ include:
   a) Solar/*Actinic keratosis*
   b) Ionizing radiation-induced keratosis
   c) Arsenical keratosis
   d) *Bowen's disease* (a solitary lesion as a slowly enlarging erythematous plaque with a sharp border, slight scaling, and some crusting); related to exposure to solar irradiation or topical arsenic.
   e) *HPV* (certain subtypes)

2. *Hyperkeratosis* is an important feature of SCC; may see ulceration with a necrotic base.

3. Any persistent nodule, plaque, or ulcer, ***especially if to*** sun-exposed areas or to the lips/at areas of radiodermatitis/in old burn scars/to the genitalia should be examined for SCC.

4. Carry a much **greater risk of metastasizing** than does basal cell ca

A Summary of Common HPV Types and Clinical Findings				
Mucosal			**Cutaneous**	
6,11	Genital warts	1	Plantar warts
34,40,42	Anogenital warts Intraepithelial neoplasia	2	Common warts
72,73	Oral papillomas in immunosuppressed pts	3	Flat warts
16,18,31,33	Anogenital malignancies	5,8	Benign warts *Squamous cell carcinoma*
		36	Actinic keratoses
		48	*Squamous cell ca*
		49	Warts, actinic keratoses

BASAL CELL CA ✪

1. The ***most common*** type of skin ca
2. Nodular or ulcerative types with ***"pearly", "rolled-up" borders***
3. Malignant in its locally aggressive growth properties, but with ***limited capacity to metastasize***.
4. ***Sun exposure*** is important in the development of this ca; arsenic exposure may also predispose.

LICHEN PLANUS

1. Flat-topped, violaceous, shiny, pruritic papules
2. Induced by drugs; examples of drugs that cause…
   a) ACE inhibitors
   b) Gold
   c) TCN
   d) Antimalarials
   e) Penicillamine
   f) Color film developer
   g) Thiazides
   h) Chlorpropamide
3. Treatment is removal of offending drug, and giving a regimen of steroids ± cyclosporine.

MEDICAL CONDITIONS ASSOCIATED WITH PRURITIS:
1. Obstructive jaundice (e.g. PBC)
2. Chronic renal failure
3. P. Vera
4. Hodgkin's; CLL
5. Hyper- and Hypothyroidism
6. Estrogens (pregnancy, OCPs)
7. Parasites
8. Drugs (e.g. narcotics)

✪ IMMUNOLOGIC MECHANISMS OF DRUG-INDUCED SKIN REACTIONS

1. **Type I** reaction (immediate hypersensitivity): <u>**Urticaria**</u> commonly caused by…
   a) PCN; Sulfonamides
   b) ASA
   c) Contrast media

2. **Type II** reaction (cytotoxic): e.g. <u>**Thrombocytopenic purpura (ITP)**</u>—commonly caused by:
   a) Methyldopa
   b) Gold

3. **Type III** reaction (vaculitis): e.g. <u>**Drug-induced lupus**</u>—commonly caused by…
   a) Hydralazine, procainamide
   b) Sulphonamides
   c) PCN

4. **Type IV** reaction (delayed, cell-mediated hypersensitivity): <u>**Contact dermatitis**</u>→Test with *<u>Patch testing</u> (not to be confused with Prick testing, which is used to investigate respiratory allery to pollens and molds)*; common causes include…

   a) **Nickle→jewelry**
   b) **Paraphenylenediamine→hair dyes/*cosmetics***
   c) **PABA→sunscreens** (immunologically related to (b) above)
   d) **Potassium Dichromate→cement, leathers, certain paints**
   e) **Formaldehyde→*cosmetics*/shampoos**
   f) **Parabens→*cosmetics***
   g) **Neomycin**
   h) **Thiuram→wearing shoes containing rubber**

DISTINGUISHING FEATURES OF THE STEVENS-JOHNSON SYNDROME
1. Systemic illness (fever, arthralgias)
2. Purulent conjuctivitis often associated with corneal ulceration/perforation
3. Buccal ulceration and bullous stomatitis ± genital/anal ulcers
4. Acute (or recurrent) bloodstained crusting of swollen lips

CONDITIONS PREDISPOSING TO AMPICILLIN RASH:
1. EBV
2. CMV
3. CLL
4. Concurrent allopurinol treatment

URTICARIA

1. **Ordinary** urticaria—may be IgE-mediated or non-immunologically-mediated (certain histamine-containing foods, like frozen tuna)
2. **Chronic** urticaria
   a) Defined as recurrent lesions for 3 months ± arthralgias, adenopathy, abdominal pain
   b) Mediated by histamine, *not* IgE; prick tests negative
   c) Steroids contraindicated
3. **Cold** urticaria—*familial form*
   a) Rash appears several hours after cold exposure
   b) Associated with fever, arthralgias, and leukocytosis
4. **Cold** urticaria—*acquired form*
   • Rash appears several minutes after skin exposure to cold water or ice
5. **Solar** urticaria
   a) Weal occurs within 30 seconds-3 minutes of sun exposure
   b) DDx includes SLE and drug photosensitivity
   c) Localized to sun-exposed areas
6. **Pressure** urticaria
   a) Affects feet, buttocks, back
   b) Tender swelling occurs 2-12 hours after pressure injury
7. **Scratch** urticaria (delayed dermatographism)
   a) Redness, weal, and itch occur hours after scratching
   b) As opposed to simple dermatographism, which affects 5% of the population and is *not* pruritic.
8. **Vasculitic** urticaria
   a) Can be life-threatening
   b) Painful, non-pruritic lesions usually lasting >24 hours
   c) ± Fever, arthralgias, abdom pain, glomerulonephritis (don't confuse with HSP, Henoch-Schonlein Purpura)
   d) ↓ Complement levels

9. **Angioneurotic edema** ✪
   ⇒Affects mucocutaneous junctions: lips/eyes/penis
   ⇒Large tender swellings, often pruritic
   ⇒Glottal edema may complicate, esp if angioedema occurs in the context of anaphylaxis
   ⇒Note that **urticaria does not occur in HANE**
   [*Hereditary* AngioNeurotic Edema, 2° to *C1 INH deficiency (C1 inhibitor)*]

PAGET'S DISEASE OF THE NIPPLE

1. Erythematous, scaly, weeping, eczematous eruption of the areola

2. Associated with underlying ductal ca of the breast

MELANOMA

◆ Most important prognosticator is **tumor thickness!** **(Breslow level)**

◆ **5 SIGNS OF MALIGNANT MELANOMA...**

Asymmetry

Border is irregular—edges irregularly scalloped

Color—mottled (haphazard display of colors); may include shades of brown, black grey, red, and white

Diameter—greater than 6.0mm (roughly the size of a pencil eraser)

Enlargement—the patient's history of an ↑ in the size of the lesion

◆ **RISK FACTORS**

Greatly ↑ risk...
1. Changing "mole" (from patient's history)
2. Presence of one or more atypical nevi or "dysplastic nevi" along with a family history of melanoma (mutations in p16 have been identified in up to half of such patients)

Moderatly ↑ risk...
1. One family member with melanoma (parent, sibling, child)
2. Sporadic dysplastic nevi
3. Congenital melanocytic nevi (risk directly proportional to size)

Slightly ↑d risk...
1. White skin, but especially poorly tanning skin
2. Red hair
3. Freckling
4. History of severe sunburn(s) as child

◆ **STAGES of Malignant Melanoma**

Stage I → Cutaneous lesion; no lymph nodes yet

Stage II → Lymph nodes now involved

Stage III→Distant mets

> ✪ *Not to be confused with the above 6mm (!), you should know that the best independent predictor of survival is the thickness of the melanoma on biopsy, and that thickness you hope is ≤.76mm for high chance of survival.*

♦ Re: **Moh's surgery** is both diagnostic and therapeutic and involves essentially shaving off the lesion tier by tier until the margins are clear per the pathologist. Melanoma is not the only indication for Moh's surgery, which can be used in tumors involving cosmetically or aesthetically sensitive zones.

♦ Remember **sentinel lymph node mapping** is used for melanoma and is increasingly being used for breast ca (to spare the patient unnecessarily extensive lymph node dissections).

AUTOIMMUNE BULLOUS DISEASES ✪

BULLOUS PEMPHIGOID	vs.	**PEMPHIGUS VULGARUS**
Relatively benign		Can be life-threatening
IgG at *basement membrane*		IgG at *intercellular substance*
Titre of circulating IgG *does not* correlate with dz activity		Titre of IgG correlates to dz activity
Tense bullae		*Flaccid* bullae
Subepidermal		Intraepidermal
Tx: *less* immunosuppressive than PV		Tx: *more* immunosuppressive than BP

> ♦ **DERMATITIS HERPETIFORMIS**—Another autoimmune bullous disease; associated with **Celiac Disease**; re: can check **anti-endomysial Ab** and **anti-gliadin Ab** to confirm the diagnosis, but don't forget the diagnostic significance of a gluten-free diet (in celiac disease)! Immunofluorescent staining is less important in this bullous disease.

DIFFERENTIAL DIAGNOSIS OF PALPABLE PURPURA

1. Vasculitis…
   a) Hypersensitivity Vasculitis (Henoch-Schonlein Purpura, or HSP, is a type of HV associated with Ig A)
   b) Septic Vasculitis (ricketssial spotted fevers)
   c) Cryoglobulinemia
   d) Wegener's, PAN, Kawasaki disease

2. TTP

3. Acute Meningococcemia (DIC with Purpura Fulminans)

4. Disseminated Gonococcemia

DERMATOLOGY

DDX OF DISCRETE HYPOPIGMENTED AREAS:
1. **Vitiligo**; *causes...*
    a) Hypo and hyperthyroidism
    b) Addison's or Cushing's
    c) SLE
    d) Alopecia Areata
2. **Tinea Versicolor** (Pityriasis Versicolor)
3. Tuberculoid Leprosy
4. **"Ash-leaf" spots of tuberous sclerosis**
5. **Morphea** (localized patches of scleroderma)

DIAGNOSTIC SIGNIFICANCE OF FINGERNAIL EXAMINATION ✪

1. **Clubbing** →TB; bronchiectasis; lung ca; COPD

2. **Pitting**→**P**soriasis; alopecia areata

3. **Subungal splinter hemorrhages**→Infective endocarditis

4. **Telangiectasia, nailfold infarts**→ Collagen-vascular diseases

5. **"Half-and-half" (Terry's) nails**→ CHF; ↓ *Albumin associated with cirrhosis*

6. **Koilonychia (spoon nails)**→Chronic Fe deficiency

7. **Onycholysis** (separation of the nail plate from the bed)→Thyrotoxicosis (esp when it affects only the ring finger); otherwise it can be seen in onychomycosis, trauma, and psoriasis

---

AND (as they say on Broadway) →"DON'T FORGET YOUR LINES"...

8. **Muehrcke's lines**→*Hypoalbuminemia associated with nephrotic syndrome.*

9. **Mee's lines (white bands)**→Arsenic poisoning

10. **Beau's lines** (Transverse furrows or ridges of the nail plate that develop after dz or chemo and caused by temporary arrest of nail plate function

HERE'S THE ERYTHEMAS AND THEIR CLINICAL SIGNIFICANCE ✪
1. E. **Nodosum**→see associated conditions below

2. E. **Chronicum Migrans (ECM)**→Lyme Disease

3. E. **Marginatum**→transient truncal rash in Rheumatic Fever

4. E. **Multiforme**-Stephen Johnson Syndrome (e.g.Dilantin, Sulfa, PCN, HSV, Mycoplasma)

5. E. **Gyratum Repens** (looks like the grain pattern of wood)→Internal malignancy (e.g. breast ca);

6. **Necrolytic Migratory Erythema (NME)**→Glucagonoma

ERYTHEMA NODOSUM ✪ ---ASSOC'D CONDITIONS → "L.U.M.P.S." (or "BLUMPYS")

L ofgren's syndrome; Lymphoma

U lcerative Colitis; Crohn's

M TB; mycoses

P arasites, **P**ills (OCPs)

S ulphonamides, Strep pharyngitis, Sarcoidosis

+ **Behcet's** (defined as recurrent painful oral ulcers plus any 2 of the following: Ocular lesions; Skin lesions; Genital ulcers; and Pathergy test); + **Yersinia** enterocol.

DISTINGUISHING PORPHYRIA CUTANEA TARDA FROM PSEUDOPORPHYRIA		
Feature	**PCT**	**Pseudoporphyria**
Abnormal porphyrin metabolism	Yes	No
Blisters on hands & face	Yes	No
Hyperpigmentation	Yes	No
Hypertrichosis	Yes	No
Milia	Yes	No
Sclerodermoid changes	Yes	No
Skin fragility	Yes	Yes
Associated conditions	SLE Hemochromatosis Hepatic tumors Hepatitis	Renal dialysis Tanning bed use
Associated drugs	Barbiturates Estrogen Ethanol Iron	Amiodarone Bumetadine Chlorthalidone Furosemide Nalidixic acid NSAIDs Retinoids TCN

So, essentially, **pseudoporphyria** is a vesiculobullous cutaneous condition that *clinically and histologically resembles several of the features of PCT but is devoid of biochemical porphyrin abnormalities.* Enhanced skin fragility and bullae formation on sun-exposed skin surfaces are the prominent features of pseudoporphyria. {*In contrast to PCT*, the presence of milia, hypertrichosis, alteration of pigmentation, sclerodermatous changes, and photo-onycholysis is generally lacking.} Lesions are usually asymptomatic.

8. NEUROLOGY AND GERIATRICS

Commonly Asked Material:

1. Recognize the clinical presentation of **acoustic neuroma** (schwannomas involving the 8th cranial nerve which grow slowly and produce hearing loss and tinnitus as most common symptoms).

2. Know the triad of **Meniere's Disease** is vertigo, tinnitus, and hearing loss that is progressive and sensorineural. 30% are bilateral. You need not have all three to make the diagnosis, but the vertigo *must* be present.

3. 2-3 questions re: patients with **recurrent unilateral CVA** and the need for inspecting/repairing the contralateral carotid a.

4. Recognize a case of **isolated peroneal neuropathy** (foot drop, etc)

5. Recognize a case of **3rd nerve palsy**. Remember: (LR6SO4)3 ; 3rd nerve is to the medial rectus.

6. **Multiple Sclerosis** (2 questions): secondary to inflammatory demyelination (which later scars to form a plaque) in the white matter of the brain (most frequently periventricular), brain stem, or spinal cord. This can lead to an otherwise healthy person presenting with exacerbations and remissions of any combination of the following symptoms: opthalmoplegia/unilateral loss of vision/diplopia/vertigo/ataxia/dysathria/paresthesias/paralysis/emotional lability.

7. Remember(B→O→M):   Botulin→presynaptic
    Organophosphate poisoning→synaptic
    Myasthenia Gravis→postsynaptic.

8. Botulism: **Remember the 6 D's →**

    Eyes→   **D ilated, fixed pupil**
    D iplopia

    Tongue→ **D ysarthria**
    D ysphagia
    D ry tongue

    And...   **D escending paralysis**

9. Recognize **Myasthenia Gravis** (often heralded by such cranial nerve findings as diplopia; dysarthria; dysphagia; dyspnea; and fatiguability) and DDx it from **Eaton Lambert** (often associated with small cell lung ca; proximal muscle weakness); also know that **Thymoma**→10% develop Myasthenia Gravis. Tensilon test for dx. Physostigmine or pyridostigmine for treatment.

10. **Guillain-Barre Syndrome**:
    - Half the patients have mild respiratory or GI infection 1-3 weeks prior
    - Severe rapidly progressive, symmetrical polyneuropathy with pronounced proximal muscle weakness; resp weakness critical (don't forget to check Negative Inspiratory Pressures and Vital Capacities frequently)

11. Know **indications for MRI**: for example:
    - Cancer patient with back pain and neuro symptoms
    - Patient with neural claudication (back pain worse with walking, etc)
    - Percussion tenderness over spine in a suspected septic discitis as well as paraspinal abscess.
    - Know that pain is the most common initial presenting symptom in cancer patients with imminent cord compression.
    - Cases of suspected avascular necrosis, e.g. of the femoral head in patients on chronic steroids, sickle cell patients, etc.

12. Recognize a case of **Diabetic Amyotrophy** → weakness, atrophy, and pain affecting the pelvic girdle and thigh muscles [it's all in the name: "a...trophy" of the "myo"(muscles)]

13. **Polymyalgia Rheumatica**: elderly patient with aching/pain and stiffness of neck/upper back/shoulders/upper arms/hip girdle; can see fever; anorexia; weight loss; Remember: no muscle weakness (that's myositis!)

14. Recognize a case of **Meralgia Paresthetica**. This is the most common pure sensory mononeuropathy, resulting from compression of the lateral cutaneous nerve of the thigh as it passes through the inguinal ligament. It presents with numbness or burning sensation over the lateral thigh; sometimes, prolonged standing or walking can provoke the symptoms. Weight loss can help, but in many cases, its spontaneously subsides.

15. Classic case of **Normal Pressure Hydrocephalus**(triad of ataxia, dementia, and incontinence)

16. **Seizures**. Know EEG indications: e.g. they present an anxious pt who seizes while getting his blood drawn; another patient who seizes after a night of dancing. Know that seizure disorder is a clinical not an EEG diagnosis and that a normal EEG does not R/O seizure disorder. Similarly brain death is a clinical diagnosis; EEG is simply an adjuvant tool in the diagnosis. Know also that Head Trauma is chief cause of focal sz in young adults, as opposed to brain tumor/vascular dz in older patients. Know that Valproic Acid may cause neural tube defects and that Tegretol/Dilantin/Phenobarb can all make OCPs less effective.

17. Similarly, in **anticonvulsant blood levels**, remember:
    - Therapeutic levels represent only average bell-shaped curves.
    - Anticonvulsant dose should never be changed based on blood levels alone.
    - Toxicity is a clinical, not a laboratory, phenomenon.

18. Recognize a classic case of **Pseudotumor Cerebri**: high opening pressure on LP; MS changes; fundoscopic changes; etc.
    - Lumbar puncture is dangerous and contraindicated when papilledema is due to *intracranial mass*, but is safe in pseudotumor cerebri.

19. Recognize a case of **Classic Migraine** and **Migraine Equivalent**.
    - *Classic Migraine*: N/V; photophobia; visual (scintillations, scotomas) and paresthetic (manual, perioral) neurologic symptoms prior to H/A.
    - *Migraine Equivalent*: recurrent attacks of neurologic dysfunction that mimic the migraine alone, but do not culminate in headache.
    - Remember, migraines (and cluster H/As) are typically unilateral, as opposed to tension H/As, which can be either unilateral or bilateral
    - *Cluster headaches*: severe; unilateral; often at the same time each day assoc'd with at least one of the following: conjunctival injection; lacrimation; nasal congestion; rhinorrhea; forehead/facial swelling; miosis; ptosis; eyelid edema. They occur qod to 8x/d over a 3-6 week period (and therefore the name).

20. **Essential tremor**: be able to DDx it from Parkinson's tremor:
    - Essential Tremor: hands/head/voice tremor→can treat with propranol or even a bit of ETOH.
    - Parkinson's Tremor: there's no head involvement.

21. Know that **Subarachnoid Hemorrhage** can present with meningismus and and incomplete 3rd nerve palsy (secondary to aneurysmal expansion); in up to 50% of cases, alert patients with aneurysm may have a small sentinel bleed with warning headache.

22. Recognize a case of **ALS (Amyotrophic Lateral Sclerosis)**: *tongue fasciculations*; weakness; atrophy; progressive limb weakness affecting distal more than proximal areas and esp affecting the small muscles of the hand; upper and lower motor neuronal involvement. Characteristically, bowel and bladder functions remain unaffected.

NEUROLOGY NOTES

LACUNAR SYNDROMES AND SITES OF ORIGIN:

Lacunar Syndrome	Usual Site of Infarct
Pure motor hemiparesis	Posterior internal capsule, corona radiata
Pure sensory CVA	Thalamus
Ataxic hemiparesis	Pons, posterior internal capsule or corona radiata
Clumsy hand dysarthria	Pons
Sensorimotor CVA	Posterior internal capsule and thalamus

CARDIOEMBOLIC SOURCES OF ISCHEMIC CVA

Major Risk Factors	Minor Risk Factors
A Fib	MVP
Mitral Stenosis	Severe mitral annular calcification
Prosthetic valve	Patent foramen ovale
Recent MI	Atrial septal aneurysm
LV thrombus	Calcific AS
Atrial myxoma	LV regional wall abnormalities
Infectious endocarditis	
Nonischemic dilated cardiomyopathy	
Nonbacterial thrombotic endocarditis	
Sick sinus syndrome	

DIFFERENTIATING ANTERIOR VS. POSTERIOR CIRCULATION CVA BY SYMPTOMS

Anterior Circulation	Posterior Circulation
Motor dysfunction (contralateral face & extremities) <ul><li>Clumsiness</li><li>Weakness</li><li>Paralysis</li><li>Slurred speach</li></ul>	Motor dysfunction (ipsilateral face; contralateral extremities) <ul><li>Clumsiness</li><li>Weakness</li><li>Paralysis</li></ul>
Loss of vision in ipsilateral eye; Homonymous hemianopia	Loss of vision in one or both homonymous visual fields
Aphasia (dominant hemisphere)	Typical signs but nondiagnostic in isolation <ul><li>Ataxia (gait or extremities)</li><li>Vertigo</li><li>Diplopia</li><li>Dysphagia</li><li>Dysarthria</li></ul>
Sensory deficity (contralateral face & extremities) <ul><li>Numbness or loss of sensation</li><li>Paresthesias</li></ul>	Sensory deficity (ipsilateral face, contralateral extrems) <ul><li>Numbness or loss of sensation</li><li>Paresthesias</li></ul>

- **Remember, in acute CVA, MRI is better for detecting ischemic CVA, while CT picks up acute hemorrhage much better.**

Causes of Continued Clinical Deterioriation Following an Apparently Completed CVA

1. Continued Emboli
2. Extension of infarct
3. Hemorrhage into infarct
4. Worsening cerebral vasospasm/edema
5. Improper diagnosis (e.g. vasculitis or tumor)

CHARACTERISTICS OF HYPERTENSIVE & DIABETIC RETINOPATHY ✪

HTN	DM
AV nicking	*Neovascularization (new vessel formation)*
Papilledema	*Microaneuysms*
Flame hemorrhages	*Dot and blot hemorrhages*
Silver/copper wiring	*Hard exudates (lipid deposits)*
	Soft exudates (cotton wool spots)

DDX OF HORNER'S SYNDROME

1. Lateral medullary syndrome
2. Pancoast tumor
3. Shy-Drager syndrome
4. Sympathectomy
5. Syringomyelia

PTOSIS

1. Complete unilateral→3rd nerve palsy
2. Partial unilateral
   a) Horner's syndrome (ptosis, meiosis, anhydrosis)
   b) Congenital (#1 cause in the healthy adult)
   c) Partial 3rd nerve palsy

3. Bilateral→muscle disease
   a) Myotonic Dystrophy
   b) Myasthenia Gravis

RAMSAY-HUNT SYNDROME

1. Varicella-zoster of the geniculate ganglion of CN 7
2. **May see *herpetic vesicles in the external ear* canal (classic), + TM involvement/vertigo/nystagmus/deafness/facial paralysis**

LATERALIZATION IN NYSTAGMUS AND CONJUGATE DEVIATION

a. *Nystagmus*
- **Vestibular lesion**→nystagmus is greatest on looking *away from* the lesion
- **Cerebellar lesion**→nystagmus is greatest on looking *towards* the lesion.

b. *Conjugate Deviation*
- **Hemispheric stroke**→eyes deviate *towards* the side of the lesion (and away from the hemiplegic extremity/ies)
- **Epileptogenic focus during seizure**→eyes deviate *away from* the side of the nidus.
- **Brainstem disease**→eyes deviate *away from* side of lateral pontine lesion (and toward the hemiplegic extremity/ies)
- **Caloric testing** in patients with intact brainstem/labyrinth→Eyes deviate *towards* the ear that is irrigated with the cold water.

> Remember, **nystagmus** from **central** causes is *vertical*. **Peripheral** etiologies lead to *horizontal or rotational* nystagmus.

SOME IMPORTANT CONSIDERATIONS IN FACIAL PAIN W/ A TRIGEMINAL DISTRIBUTIONS

a. **Trigeminal Neuralgia**
- Generally seen in patients > 50yo
- The pain commonly involves the *maxillary and mandibular* branches of the fifth cranial nerve.

b. **Intracavernous Internal Carotid Artery Aneurysm**
- May lead to opthalmoplegia, esp CN III
- Sensory loss/pain to the *opthalmic ± maxillary* branches of CN V

c. **Post-herpetic neuralgia**
- Most common among the elderly
- Pain in the *opthalmic* branch of CN V

PHYSICAL EXAM IN HEARING LOSS

Methods

> 1. **Weber's Test**→Tests using lateralization
> 2. **Rinne's Test** →Tests using conduction differences

INTERPRETING WEBER'S TEST

1. Lateralizes to deaf side in *conduction deafness* (e.g. otosclerosis)
2. Lateralizes to normal side in *nerve deafness* (e.g. acoustic neuroma)

INTERPRETING RINNE'S TEST

1. Bone conduction > Air conduction on the affected side in *conduction deafness*
2. Air conduction > Bone conduction on both sides in *nerve deafness*

OR, (if you really like misery)…

Rinne Test
- Holding the tuning fork against the mastoid process, the patient indicates when s/he can no longer hear the sound. At that point the tuning fork is changed to just outside the auditory meatus to see if the sound can be heard again. *Normal hearing patients and patients with sensorineural hearing loss* hear the sound longer through air than through bone, noted as "AC>BC" (air conduction > bone conduction). In a *conductive hearing loss*, bone conduction becomes ≥ air conduction, **paradoxically**. This results is reported as an "abnormal Rinne" or "reversed Rinne".

Weber Test
- Holding the tuning fork on the middle of the patient's forhead, the patient is asked, "Where do you hear this the loudest?" The sound **localizes** *toward the side with conducting loss (toward the worse-hearing ear) or away from the side with a sensorineural loss (toward the better hearing ear).* The Weber test is only useful if there is an asymmetric hearing loss. If hearing is symmetric, the patient perceives the sound in the middle of the forehead.

UPPER MOTOR NEURON Lesions	**vs.**	**LOWER MOTOR NEURON Lesions**
↑ Tone ± clonus		↓ Tone
↑ DTRs		↓ DTRs
Babinski (extensor plantar response)		No Babinski
Absent abdomenal reflexes		
		Fasciculations
		Atrophy

Reflex (DTR) present?	→	**Nerve Root Intact**
Biceps (supinator jerk present)		C6
Triceps reflex		C8
Abdominal reflex		T7-12
Cremasteric reflex		L1/2
Patellar reflex		L3/4
Achilles reflex		S1
Anal reflex		S3/4

- If you see **unilateral wasting of the small hand muscles**, think of either an *ulnar nerve* lesion or a *T1 nerve root* lesion, such as might be caused by a bronchogenic carcinoma.

✪ **Peripheral Neuropathy**   →   **CN involvement**
Diabetes   CN 3,4,6
Guillain-Barre   CN 6,7
Sarcoidosis   CN 7
Diptheria   CN 9

✪ **Aneurysm**   →   **CN involvement**
ICA at the cavernous sinus   CN 3-6
Opthalmic artery   CN 2
PCA (post communicating)   CN 6

DETERMINATION OF BRAIN DEATH
1. Sufficient cause—must exclude hypothermia and sedative overdose
2. Absent gag/corneal/cough reflexes
3. Fixed pupils
4. Loss of oculovestibular and oculocephalic reflexes
5. No response to painful stimuli, except for spinal reflexes
6. No spontaneous respiratory movements after ventilator disconnected and patient observed for 5 minutes with oxygen supplied via tracheal catheter.

DIAGNOSTIC LIMITATIONS OF THE EEG
1. Cannot exclude epilepsy
2. Cannot exclude focal pathology
3. Cannot suggest structural nature of focal pathology
4. Cannot be used to assess the adequacy of antiseizure medication
5. In determining brain death, if brain stem reflexes are present OR if they are persistently absent, there is no need to order an EEG.

✪ INTERPRETIVE PATTERNS IN EMG (ELECTROMYOGRAPHY)

1. Myasthenia Gravis→*__decremental response__* to repetitive ('tetanic') stimulation

2. Myasthenic syndrome (**Eaton-Lambert Syndrome**)→ *__Incremental response__* to such stimulation

3. Myotonia→**'Dive-bomber'** EMG (*high frequency* action potential discharges)

4. Polymyositis→**Fibrillation** (brief *low-amplitude* action potentials due to 'denervation hypersensitivity' at the motor end plate)

✪ On exam, **ELS can be differentiated from Myasthenia Gravis** since ELS patients derive ↑ strength from repeated activity, while Myasthenic patients get weaker.

WHEN IS IT APPROPRIATE TO MONITOR ANTICONVULSANT LEVELS?

1. Suspect non-compliance
2. Renal or hepatic disease
3. Poor seizure control
4. Suspected toxicity
   a) **Phenytoin**
      (1) Gingival hyperplasia
      (2) Hirsutism
      (3) Nystagmus →ataxia→drowsiness
      (4) Osteomalacia
      (5) Arrthmias/Hypotension in IV use
   b) **Carbamazepine**
      (1) Drowsiness (esp if used with phenytoin)
      (2) Leukopenia
      (3) SIADH
      (4) Anticholinergic effects (structurally similar to tricyclics)
   c) **Valproic Acid**
      (1) Tremor
      (2) Hair Thinning
      (3) ↑appetite/weight gain; ankle edema

   - *Note all 3 of the above may cause drowsiness and ataxia*

5. 2nd drug added which could potentiate or diminish its activity.

CONDITIONS PREDISPOSING TO CEREBRAL ANEURYSMS

1. Polycystic Kidney Disease
2. Essential HTN
3. Aortic Coarctation
4. Ehlers-Danlos Syndrome
5. Renal Artery Stenosis due to FMD (fibromuscular dysplasia)
6. Wegener's/PAN/SBE

PREDOMINANT VERTEBRAL LEVELS IN SPECIFIC DISORDERS

Cervical Cord
   - Syringomyelia
   - Siphylitic myelitis

Thoracic Cord
   - Anterior spinal artery thrombosis
   - Pott's disease (TB)
   - Subacute Combined Degeneration (B12 deficiency)

Thoracolumbar
   - Transverse Myelitis
   - Metastases

Lumbosacral
   - Tabes Dorsalis

DIAGNOSTIC INVESTIGATION IN MYASTHENIA GRAVIS ✪

1. **Tensilon test** (Edrophonium)—should improve the symptoms, but is very short acting.
2. EMG→should see a _decremental response to repetitive stimulation ('post-tetanic inhibition')_
3. **Acetylcholine receptor Antibodies**—bear a 90% sensitivity (70% in ocular myasthenia)

Parkinson's Disease (SMART)...

S huffling gait

M asked facies

A kinesia

R igidity (cogwheel)

T remor

POINTS TO REMEMBER WITH PARKINSON'S DISEASE

- PD is a **clinical** diagnosis
- Drug therapy should be initiated only when symptoms have a negative impact on the patient's ability to function.
- **Levodopa (L-Dopa)** is the most effective drug for PD; it is used in combination with carbidopa
- Several **dopamine antagonists** are available. They are somewhat less effective than L-Dopa but are less prone to induce dyskinesias. A patient's failure to respond to one dopamine antagonist does not mean that s/he will not benefit from another.
- **Tolcapone**, one of the newer agents, inhibits dopa metabolism in plasma and allows higher amounts of L-Dopa to cross the blood-brain barrier without increasing the L-Dopa dose.
- **Anticholinergics** are the oldest group of PD medications and most effective in persons with tremor-predominant disease.
- Consider **surgery** for the patient only after medical therapies fail to confer benefit. Palliative surgeries, such as pallidotomy and thalamic deep brain stimulator implantation as well as so-called "restorative" surgeries, such as fetal mesencephalic cell transplantation are a few of the surgical options available to such individuals.

VERTIGO

- ◆ _Vestibular neuronitis_ is felt to be 2° to viral infection to the vestibular nerve/ vestibular apparatus and usually lasts a few weeks

- ✪ _BPV_ (Benign Positional Vertigo) is a vertigo brought about by specific head positions and the most common presenting complaint is vertigo on _rolling over in bed_, e.g. in getting out of bed in the morning, and _turning the head_, e.g. while changing lanes.

- ◆ _Labyrinthitis_ may be the result of bacterial or viral infection.

- ◆ _Vestibular ototoxicity (2° drugs)_ is usually a more chronic condition, accompanied by disequilibrium and hearing loss.

DDX OF VERTIGO

Central
1. Basilar Migraine
2. Cerebellopontine angle neoplasm
3. Multiple Sclerosis
4. Posterior fossa tumor
5. Vertebrobasilar ischemia

Peripheral
1. Medications
2. Motion sickness
3. Benign Positional Vertigo (BPV)
4. Vestibular Neuronitis
5. Labyrinthitis
6. Meniere's Disease
7. Trauma

UNDERSTANDING TERMS IN ABNORMAL MOTOR KINETICS:

Movement	Tone	Rate	Description	Miscellaneous
Ballism	0	Rapid	Abrupt, irregular, large amplitude	Proximal muscle
Chorea	1+	Rapid	Jerky, irregular, no rhythm	Distal muscle; semi-purposeful
Athetosis	3+	Slow	Snake-like/writhing	Digits/hands/tongue; purposeless
Cogwheel rigidity	5+	N/A	Intermittent, unintentional resistance to passive motion	Commonly seen in Parkinson's Disease

PROGRESSIVE SUPRANUCLEAR PALSY ✪
1. A key differential in Parkinson's Disease
2. It resemble Parkinson's in most ways, except :
   a) There is usually no resting tremor in SNP
   b) Patients with SNP can have a vertical gaze palsy, particularly on downward gaze, so often present with frequent falls.

CLINICAL FEATURES OF COMMON TREMORS			
Feature	**Essential**	**Parkinsonian**	**Cerebellar**
Best seen	With certain postures	At rest	With action
Frequency (cycles/s)	4-12	4-6	3-5
Aggravated by	Stress, anxiety	Stress, walking	Action
Relieved by	Alcohol	Action	Rest
Associated features	Voice, head, chin tremors	Rigidity, bradykinesia, gait	Dysarthria, ataxia, nystagmus
Disabling	Can be	Unusual	Yes
Common Cause	Familial	Idiopathic	Various

MULTIPLE SCLEROSIS

1. Consider MS when patient presents with periodic alterations in vision (e.g. central vision blurring), as well as sensory-motor skills.
2. Common optic findings include
   a) Diplopia (usually 2° to INO, or internuclear opthalmoplegia)
   b) Optic neuritis (pain on ocular movement)
   c) Nystagmus
3. Patients frequently note ↑ exacerbations in hot weather
4. Diagnosis is usually made when clinical suspicion leads to an MRI, which shows plaques in the white matter, esp the periventricular white matter; corpus callosum is a frequent site of involvement.
5. *Oligoclonal bands* are seen on CSF examination.

KEY SYMPTOMS
   ♦ Bowel/bladder/sexual dysfunction
   ♦ Cognitive Deficits
   ♦ Depression
   ♦ Fatigue
   ♦ Impaired mobility
   ♦ Pain
   ♦ Sensory changes
   ♦ Spasticity
   ♦ Speech/swallowing trouble
   ♦ Tremor
   ♦ Visual Changes
   ♦ Weakness

CLAUDICATION-2 TYPES ✪

Diagnosis	Achieves Relief With...
1) Neurogenic (pseudoclaudication)(spinal stenosis)	Sitting down/lean forward
2) Vascular	Standing still

SIGNS AND SYMPTOMS OF INCREASED INTRACRANIAL PRESSURE

1. Throbbing intermittent pain
2. Nausea and vomiting
3. Visual impairment
4. Papilledema
5. Decreased level of consciousness
6. Abnormal gait
7. Lateral rectus paresis

DIAGNOSTIC FEATURES OF HEADACHES

Migraine *without* Aura (aka *Common* Migraine)

- Pain distribution predominantly on one side of the head
- Pulsating and throbbing quality to the pain
- Moderate to severe intensity
- Sensitivity to light and sound
- Durations typically 4-72h if untreated
- Similar headaches in the past

Migraine *with* Aura (aka *Classic* Migraine)

- As above, plus an aura (visual warning of scintillating scotomata or fortification spectra)
- Aura duration typically < 60 min
- Aura onset typically 1-2 h before the H/A
- Alternatively, aura alone without subsequent H/A development (acephalgic migraine or migraine equivalent)

Prodromal Symptoms of Migraine With Aura	
Clinical descriptor	**What it Actually Means**
"Alice in Wonderland" syndrome	Visual and auditory hallucinations
Fortification spectra	Zigzag pattern resembling the facade of a fort
Hemianopia	Partial visual field loss
Paresthesias	Burning, prickling, tingling, or tickling sensations
Photopsia	Flashing lights
Scotomata	Blind spots
Teichopsia	Bright shimmering or wavy lines

Episodic Tension H/A
- Distribution generally B/L
- Pressing, squeezing, or band-like (throbbing during physical exertion)
- Mild to moderate in intensity
- Sensitivity to light or sound
- No nausea
- Duration from 30min-7days
- <15 headache days/month

Chronic Tension H/A
- As above, but ≥15 headache days/month
- Nausea may be present during intense or prolonged H/A

Episodic Cluster H/A
- Severe unilateral orbital, supraorbital, or temporal pain
- Duration 15-180 min (if untreated)
- Associated with at least one ipsilateral autonomic sign: (e.g. conjunctival injection, lacrimation, nasal congestion, rhinorrhea, sweating, miosis, ptosis, or eye edema)
- Frequency of attacks from 1 QOD - 8 QD
- Cycles last from 7days to 1 year and are separated by pain-free periods lasting ≥14days

Chronic Cluster H/A
- As above, except that cycles last >1year or are separated by remissions lasting < 14 days

GERIATRICS

URINARY INCONTINENCE ✪			
Type	**Presentation**	**Associated Findings**	**Pathophysiology**
STRESS	Small amounts of leaking with stress (*coughing, sneezing, laughing,* or *physical activity* such as bending)	Multiparity; Estrogen deficiency Prior urethral procedure or radiation	*Urethral hypermobility; internal sphinctor deficiency*
URGE	*Sudden*, uncontrollable need to void resulting in loss of large amount of urine; *nocturia* and frequency also common	*Motor urgency:* CNS-related (CVA, Alzheimer's Dz, Parkinson's Dz, MS); spinal cord pathology; *Sensory urgency:* local bladder pathology or sudden ↑ in bladder volume (diuretic or glycosuria)	*Abnormal bladder contractions*; due to *detrusor instability* in a large % of these patients.
OVERFLOW	Poor stream, straining, dribbling, although may present similar to urge or stress incontinence	*Obstruction* (BPH, fecal impaction, tumor); *Chronic bladder overdistension* (such as from DM or detrusor areflexia)	**Bladder** *overdistension*

MEDS ASSOCIATED WITH URINARY INCONTINENCE:		
Class	**Mechanism of action**	**Type of incontinence**
α agonists; β blockers	↑ tone of internal sphinctor leading to *obstruction*	Overflow
α blockers	↓ tone of internal sphinctor leading to *leakage*	Stress
Anticholinergics; and Calcium channel blockers	↓ bladder *contractions*	Overflow
Diuretics	Brisk filling of the bladder	Urge
Sedatives/hynotics/opiates/alcohol	Produce confusion; ↓ bladder contractions Depress central inhibition of micturition	Functional overflow

Agents that ↓ Bladder Contractility and Are Therefore Useful in URGE Incontinence	
Agent	**Action**
ANTICHOLINERGICS (use limited by ↑side effects) • Atropine • L-Hyoscyamine • Propantheline	Antagonize muscarinic receptors of the bladder, causing relaxation
ANTICHOLINERGIC + ANTISPASMODICS • Oxybutinin (**Ditropan®, Ditropan XL®**) • Dicyclomine (Bentyl®, etc.) • Flavoxate (**Urispas®**) • Tolterodine (**Detrol®**)	Additional smooth muscle relaxing properties
TCAs (drugs of choice for *mixed incontinence*) • Amitriptylline (Elavil®) • Doxepin (Sinequan®) • Imipramine (Tofranil®)	Both anticholinergic and α-agonist effects
CCBs • Nifedipine	Relax muscles through calcium influx blockage into cells; also probably anticholinergic effect

Agents that ↑ Urethral Resistance and are Therefore Useful in __STRESS__ Incontinence:	
Agent	**Action**
α-agonists • Ephedrine • Phenylpropanolamine	Affect symp innervation to the proximal urethra, causing ↑ pressure
TCAs	Both anticholinergic and α-agonist effects
Estrogen (hormone replacement therapy)	Thought to improve vaginal and urethral vascularity and tone

THE EFFECT OF AGE ON VARIOUS LABS ✪

__↑ with Age__	__↓ with Age__	__No Effect with Age__
Alk phos	Serum albumin	Bilirubin
Uric acid	Serum Mg	AST, ALT, GGTP
Total cholesterol	PaO2	pH, PaCO2
HDL	Creat clearance	Serum creatinine
Triglycerides	T3, TSH	T4
Fasting blood glucose	WBC	Hgb, Hct, platelets, RBC indices
1h postprandial glucose	Vit B12	
2h postprandial glucose	CPK	
ESR		

✪ SLEEP PATTERNS ASSOCIATED WITH NORMAL AGING

- ◆ No change in sleep requirements

- ◆ ↑ Nocturnal awakenings

- ◆ ↑ Sleep latency

- ◆ ↓ Deep sleep

- ◆ ↓ REM sleep

- ◆ ↓ Sleep efficiency

- ◆ Advanced sleep-wake cycle (earlier bedtime and arising time)

Miscellaneous Recurring Items...

Mixed Urge/Stress Incontinence
- 1/3 of incontinent older women have _mixed urge/stress incontinence_. The most appropriate initial management is behavioral therapy with pelvic muscle exercises and bladder training.

CATARACTS
- Know that older pts with cataracts can have normal visual acuity and yet have various types of functional visual impairment, such as _nighttime glare and disorders of depth and contrast perception often associated with falls even in the face of normal visual acuity_, which is therefore inadequate to assess the total impact of a cataract on vision.

ANEMIA
- Know that the presence of mild anemia associated with low serum Fe and TIBC strongly suggests *Anemia of Chronic Disease*.

SUBCORTICAL DEMENTIAS
- e.g. Parkinson's Dz; low-pressure hydrocephalus; M.I.D (multi-infarct dementia)
- Characterized by _prominent motor_ abnormalities and by _changes in mood, personality, impulse control, and difficulty with planning._

CORTICAL DEMENTIA
- e.g. Alzheimer's Dz
- characterized by disturbances in higher cortical functions that include language, calculation, visuospatial skills, and praxis (ability to follow commands)

CAPACITY
- Recognize that patients with dementia can still make some of their own decisions, even if e.g., they may be legally incompetent to manage their own financial affairs. Patients with dementia are frequently found by physicians, nurses, and social workers to be *capable of making their own decisions*. So, for example, if you had such a patient with Advance Directives, these directives do not go into effect until he or she is no longer able to make her own decisions, so her current, expressed wishes should be adhered to, even if there is disagreement among family members.
- Remember, a person's current wishes (if pt has capacity) preempt his or her *Advance Directives*, which in turn preempt (if there is no capacity) the wishes of a previously designated *Health Care Proxy*. When all else fails and we have none of the aforementioned, the physician can exert *Substituted Judgment*.
- "Consult the hospital ethics committee" is usually not the answer. They want _you_ to know these basic principles.

MULTI-DISCIPLINARY APPROACH
- On the exam it is important to recognize this in developing a care plan early in the hospital course for a frail older person who is functionally impaired.

DELIRIUM

- ♦ Be able to recognize that the sudden change in behavior of a patient with dementia and multiple medical problems may be the onset of delirium, which requires a thorough medical evaluation.
- ♦ Remember this Mnemonic for the causes of "*DELIRIUM*": **D**rugs—**E**lectrolyte imbalance—**L**ow pCO_2—**I**nfection—**R**elapsing fever—**I**njury to brain—**U**remia— **M**etabolic (liver damage)
- ♦ Keep in mind the key differences between Cortical Dementia and Delirium:

	DEMENTIA	*DELIRIUM*
Onset	Insidious	Sudden
Duration	Chronic	Acute
Speech	OK	Slurred
Attention	OK	Impaired
Perception	OK	Hallucinations common
Mood/affect	Apathetic/loss of impulse control	Fear/suspiciousness often present

HALLUCINATIONS
- ♦ Visual—often organic in origin; e.g. delirium
- ♦ Auditory—usually inorganic in origin; think of schizophrenia

MAJOR DEPRESSION—DIAGNOSTIC CRITERIA:
- ♦ At least 5 of the following occurring each day during a 2 wk period, representing a change from previous function: (#1 or #2 is a required criterion) and not due to medication or other condition:

  1. Depressed mood most of the day
  2. Anhedonia
  3. Unintended change in weight or appetite
  4. Insomnia/Hypersomnia
  5. Psychomotor agitation/retardation
  6. Fatigue or loss of energy
  7. Feelings of worthlessness or inappropriate guilt
  8. Diminished ability to think/concentrate/make decisions
  9. Recurrent thoughts of death or suicide

REHABILITATION
- ♦ Be able to recognize the most appropriate management of hospital discharge of a severely functionally impaired older patient who need rehab to recover functional ability.
- ♦ e.g. to an extended care facility, such as a nursing home with an on-site facility or a hospital based transitional care or rehabilitation unit.
- ♦ Often the hospital's emphasis is on an expedient discharge to the first nursing home with an available bed when the patient has rehabilitation potential.

9. ALLERGY & IMMUNOLOGY

SYMPTOMS AND SIGNS OF ANAPHYLAXIS
1. Bronchospasm
2. Diffuse erythema
3. Hypotension
4. Laryngeal edema
5. Nausea & Vomiting
6. Sense of warmth
7. Urticaria/Angioedema

TREATMENT OF ANAPHYLAXIS
1. Antihistamines to block the effects of further histamine release
2. Epinephrine .3ml of 1:1000 s.c.
3. Fluids, especially plasma expanders or .5-10 ml (cardiac arrest) of 1:10,000 IVP
4. Steroids-no help for acute attack, but may diminish subsequent reactions
5. Tracheostomy, O2, Aminophylline as needed

MAIN CAUSES OF ANAPHYLACTIC REACTIONS
1. 75% due to PCN
2. 15% due to *Hymenoptera* stings (bees, yellow jackets, hornets, wasps)
3. Reactions to latex and foods account for much of the rest

- Remember, when a patient is allergic to PCN, s/he is usually allergic to the beta-lactam ring. *Other beta-lactam antibiotics* include cephalosporins, monobactams, and carbapenams.
- In patients who are allergic to PCN, approximately 5% will develop an allergic reaction if challenged with a cephalosporin.

- ✪ Main cause of *__Anaphylactoid__* reactions is *__Radiocontrast Media__* (75% of cases)
- ✪ Remember, anaphylactoid reactions resemble anaphylaxis reactions in most ways, except they are not mediated by specific Ab (e.g. Ig E)
- ✪ Because they are not mediated by IgE, skin tests are useless

---

CAUSES OF ANAPHYLACTOID REACTIONS ✪
1. Radiocontrast media
2. Medications (ASA or NSAIDs; narcotics; protamine vancomycin)
3. Dialysis
4. Physical stimuli (cold, exercise)
5. Plasma expanders
6. Transfusion reactions

RADIOCONTRAST MEDIA REACTIONS ✪

1. <u>Anaphylactoid</u> reaction 2° to high osmolality of contrast media
2. <u>No Ig E involved</u>
3. <u>No association with shellfish allergy or iodine</u>
4. If patient had a bad reaction in the past, s/he has a 20-35% risk of a similar reaction on reexposure to these media.
5. A combination of Prednisone/Diphenhydramine/Ephedrine can prevent ~90% of these reactions. Lower osmolar media are also better received.

✪ IMMUNE REACTIONS—Types I, II, III, and IV:		
Type	**Mediators**	**Examples**
I Immediate hypersensitivity (wheal-and-flare)	Specific IgE antibody	Allergic rhinitis Anaphylaxis; asthma urticaria
II Cytotoxic	Cytotoxic cells or specific Ab plus complement	Goodpasture's Graves' disease Myasthenia Gravis Immune hemolytic anemia and thrombocytopenia
III Immune complex (Arthrus rxn)	Specific IgG/M which complexes with circulating Ag and then complement	R.A.; SLE; Hep B viral prodrome
IV Delayed hypersensitivity (cell-mediated)	Specific T-cells that release lymphokines	Contact Dermatitis GVHD Response to TB/fungal/viral infections PPD testing

✪ EXAMPLES OF CONTACT DERMATITIS

- ♦ Ethylenediamine (part of aminophylline)
- ♦ K+ Dichromate (cement)
- ♦ Nail polish (e.g. eyelid dermatitis)
- ♦ Neomycin
- ♦ Nickel sulfate
- ♦ Para-phenylenediamine (hair dyes)
- ♦ Poison ivy

ATOPIC DERMATITIS
1. High IgE associated
2. Depressed cell-mediated immunity
3. Patients tend to have a significant family history of allergic-type conditions, including allergic rhinitis, asthma, and eczema.

IN ORDER TO HAVE ASTHMA, YOU NEED 3 THINGS:
1. Reversible airway obstruction (as measured by PEFR or FEV1)
2. Airway inflammation
3. Airway hyperresponsiveness

RAST Testing ✪
1. Measures specific IgE to various Ag
2. More specific, but less sensitive than skin testing, therefore RAST is indicated in those individuals who are so exquisitely sensitive to an Ag that skin testing may yield a systemic reaction.
3. RAST is also appropriate in patients who are unable to discontinue certain medications that would otherwise affect skin testing results.

USUAL ALLERGENS IN ALLERGIC RHINITIS BY TIME OF YEAR ✪		
Seasonal	**Springtime**	**Tree and grass pollen**
	Fall	**Ragweed**
Perennial		**Dustmites; animal dander; molds**

IMMUNODEFICIENCY DISEASES	
Immunologic Defect	**Clinical Examples**
B cells	• Recurrent infections with extracellular, encapsulated bacteria
	• IgA deficiency (most patients asymp; if symptomatic, may see GI or Pulm infections)
	• X-linked agammaglobulinemia
T cells	• TB, fungal, pneumocystis, toxoplasmosis infections; DiGeorge syndrome (deficient thyroid and parathyroids)
Neutrophils	• Chronic granulomatous disease; • Chediak Higashi disease
Complement Terminal components C3 C6,7 C1esterase inhibitor	• Recurrent neisseria infections • Pyogenic infections • Raynauds phenomena • Hereditary angioedema

Warning Signs and Symptoms for Urgent Opthalmologic Referral:	
Ocular Finding:	**Associated Conditions:**
Severe Eye Pain	Uveitis, scleritis, angle-closure glaucoma (ACG) microbial keratitis, iridocyclitis
Photophobia	Iridocyclitis, keratitis, ACG
Impaired vision/loss of vision	Uveitis, scleritis, ACG, microbial keratitis, iridocyclitis
Corneal abnormalities	Corneal laceration, ACG, microbial keratitis
Pupillary abnormalities	Uveitis, ACG
Anterior chamber abnormality	Intraocular foreign body, hyphema, hypopyon, corneal perforation, ACG

OTHER CONDITIONS THAT WARRANT OPTHALMOLOGIC REFERRAL:

1. Acute or chronic motility disorder
2. Central retinal artery or vein occlusion
3. Chemical or alkali burn
4. Corneal ulceration or abrasion that does not heal within 48 h
5. Diabetic retinopathy
6. Endopthalmitis
7. Herpetic corneal lesions
8. Hyphema (blood in anterior chamber)
9. Macular degeneration
10. Orbital cellulitis
11. Penetrating trauma
12. Retinal detachment

10. CARDIOLOGY PART I: ELECTROCARDIOGRAPHY PEARLS PLUS!

HERE'S THE _EASY_ WAY TO FIGURE THE AXIS!

Look at the direction of the R-wave in leads I and aVF:

	I	**aVF**
Normal axis ("2 thumbs up")	↑	↑
LAD	↑	↓
RAD	↓	↑
Extreme RAD	↓	↓

EFFECTS OF CAROTID SINUS MASSAGE OR ADENOSINE (Diagnostic And Therapeutic)
1. A tach/flutter/fib→AV block
2. PAT→Termination/NSR (Normal Sinus Rhythm)
3. Sinus Tach→Transient slowing
4. V Tach→No effect

CAUSES OF LOW-VOLTAGE EKG
1. Calibration off
2. Obesity→other tissue
3. Tamponade→pericardial space
4. Pericardial effusion→pericardial space
5. Cardiomyopathy / Myocarditis →heart
6. Global ischemia→heart
7. Breast tissue (lead placement)→other tissue

CAUSES OF TALL R-WAVE (R>S) IN V1 OR V2:
1. Dextrocardia
2. Hypertrophic cardiomyopathy
3. Posterior wall MI
4. RBBB
5. RVH
6. WPW→√ for delta wave
7. RAD (right axis deviation)→check the axis!
8. Rotation of heart (5% of population)
9. Normal variant among young females

PEARL: <u>Rhythm</u> is best read by √ing V1, except if Afib or Aflutter, when rhythm is best made out in the inferior leads, and <u>intervals</u> are best read at lead II.

PEARL: You can't read ST-T wave changes in AFib or Aflutter.

PEARL: The only time *aVR* helps is in *pericarditis* where ST depression (***"bent knee" sign***) may sometimes be found. *Beware too*: the disappearance of pain may sometimes signal a new pericardial effusion.

PEARL: A true 'pause' is defined as $\geq$ 3s between 2 adjacent R-waves.

SOME CAUSES OF PATHOLOGICAL 'Q' WAVES
1. Cardiac contusion; myocarditis
2. Hyperkalemia
3. Hypertrophic CMP
4. LBBB
5. Poor lead placement
6. Transmural MI
7. WPW

DDX OF ↑QTc (differential dx of increased <u>c</u>alculated QT interval):
1. Ischemia: #1 cause
2. ↓Mg, ↓K+, ↓Ca; ↓thyroid
3. Pentamidine
4. Tricyclic antidepressants; Phenothiazines
5. IA Antiarrythimics (e.g. PDQ: procainamide; disopyramide; quinidine)
6. Amiodarone
7. Any combination of Seldane with Erythro/Cisapride (pulled from the US market) /Azoles (e.g. ketoconazole)/Lovastatin

PEARL: QTc: Even though the 'c' stands for <u>c</u>alculated, you should really think of it as '<u>c</u>orrected' for the heart rate—because imagine the heart rate was at 300: the QT would be very short indeed! The QTc therefore takes the heartrate into account.
$\Rightarrow$ **THEREFORE,** remember the **RULE OF THUMB to recognize ↑ QTc:** If the QT interval (whatever the rate) is more than half the R-R interval, then the QT is prolonged.

- **PEARL**: ↑QTc is important because it **can progress to Torsades** (de Pointes) which can in turn progress to VT.

Remember…
- **Digoxin** can: ↑PR, and ↓QTc; but **Quinidine** can ↑ all the intervals.
- **K+ can:** 1) flatten the PR; 2) broaden the QRS; and 3) peak the 'T'-waves. In severe cases, you may see a 'sign-wave' that can progress to asystole.

ABSENT 'P' WAVES
1. A fib
2. Sino-atrial block
3. Severe ↑K+

EKG LOCALIZATION OF ACUTE INFARCTS
1. Anterior MI→Q waves/ST↑ V2-4
2. Extensive Anterior MI→ as above in I, aVL, and V1-6
3. Anteroseptal MI→Q waves/ST↑ in V1-3
4. Anterolateral MI→ Q waves/ST↑ V4-6, I, aVL
5. Inferior MI→Q waves/ST↑ II, III, aVF
6. Right Ventricular MI→ST↑ in V4R (i.e. lead V4 on right-sided lead placement)
7. Posterior MI→see next…

EKG in POSTERIOR MI
1. Tall, widened 'R' and 'T' waves in V1,2
2. Upsloping ST depression in V1,2
3. Usually associated with signs of inferior MI

HYPERACUTE T-WAVES
1. M.I.
2. ↑K+
3. Normal Variant
4. LBBB

U-WAVES
1. Follows the T wave and is inverted just like the letter "U".
2. May be a normal variant; or
3. 2° to electrolyte imbalance

POOR R-WAVE PROGRESSION
1. In general, the height of the R-wave should ↑ as one moves across the precordium from V1→V6.
2. Normally, you should see an R-wave height of 3mm by V3, or 4mm by V4
3. If V3R>V4R, that's called "regression", and that's usually evidence of infarct.
4. Beware, however, that an EKG taken during a prolonged inspiration (heart moves away from chest wall leads) can simulate this, so should repeat on normal breathing.

- **PEARL**: Remember, you always have to repeat the EKG to check for motion up or down of the ST segment (this is true also for T-wave inversion). Any movement is *usually* indicative of <u>ischemia</u>. On the other hand, *no* movement/resolution of an ST segment elevation or a T-wave inversion, given the proper scenario, may be indicative of <u>infarction</u>.

CAUSES OF AN ELEVATED ST SEGMENT
1. Pericarditis (diffuse, concave ST ↑; PR depression often noted)
2. Coronary spasm (Prinztmetal's angina, aka 'variant' angina)
3. Ventricular aneurysm
4. ↑K+
5. Ischemia
6. LVH
7. LBBB
8. Early repolarization
9. CHF

PEARL: PACs (Premature atrial contractions) have longer PR intervals than sinus beats.

ASHMAN'S PHENOMENON ("SHORT-LONG-SHORT")
- Refers to *the 3 R-R interval immediately preceding a PAC to help identify the complex as a PAC* (as opposed to a PVC), particularly in AFib or A Flutter. Remember too that a PAC has a longer PR interval than the sinus beat (2° to conduction delay).

Remember: **PACs can be an early sign of occult CHF.**

CRITERIA FOR LVH
1. R-wave in lead I ≥ 11mm
2. R-wave in aVL ≥ 12
3. S in V1/2 + R in V5/6 ≥ 35 (really any 2 precordial leads)
4. S in V2 ≥ 25
5. R in I + S in III ≥ 25

4 TYPES OF ST DEPRESSION
1. **Flat** → **ISCHEMIA**
2. **Downsloping** → **ISCHEMIA**
3. **Upsloping** → Non-specific
4. **Concave/ 'scooped-out'** → Digoxin-induced

3-MINUTE INSTANT E.R. PROGNOSTICATORS IN MI:
(all of these can be done <u>at bedside</u> and all confer a mortality *twice* those without the risk factor)

1. Age>75
2. Prior MI
3. Presence of DM
4. AFib or Aflutter
5. SBP<80
6. HR>100
7. BBB

♦ Low Ejection Fraction and a positive stress test are additional poor prognosticators following MI.

EKG PROGRESSION OF M.I.
1. First see hyperacute T-waves;
2. Then see ST ↑
3. Finally Q-waves form.

IN ORDER TO CALL RVH, ONE MUST 1st R/O
1. RBBB
2. LPHB
3. Anterolateral or IW MI

• Look for R>S in V1/2
• Look for S>R in V5/6

> If you see RVH + Pulmonary HTN in a young women→R/O ASD.

MORE PEARLS YOU HAVE TO KNOW...

• **PEARL**: If you see true **angina + ST↑** (not Printzmetal's) or if you **see angina + <u>new</u> BBB</u>→ thrombolytics** are justified in the ER setting (assuming no contraindications to thrombolytics).
♦ <u>Absolute contraindications</u> include:
   1) Prior intracranial bleed or CNS tumor;
   2) Recent prolonged CPR;
   3) Active internal bleeding;
   4) CVA or head trauma within the previous 6 months;
   5) Use of Streptokinase for the second time in a year, since patient builds up antibodies to it and tends to react poorly the second time if used so soon after.

◆ **<u>Relative contraindications</u> include:**
   1) GIB within 1 month;
   2) Surgery or trauma in the past 2 weeks;
   3) Pregnancy;
   4) BP >200/110.

- **PEARL: Remember, <u>Streptokinase</u> commonly causes <u>Hypotension</u>**

- **PEARL: For acute MI, must have <u>ST elevations</u> of <u>1mm</u> in the limb leads or <u>2mm</u> in the V (chest) leads.**

- **PEARL:** Nevertheless, always remember that *any Q-waves*—**even so-called 'baby' Q-waves, in leads <u>V1 or V2</u> are significant**.

- **PEARL: Routine/prophylactic use of Lidocaine peri-MI should not be practiced** as it can actually ↑ mortality, if used indiscriminately, and should only be used in patients who show evidence of VT.

- **PEARL:** When see **akinesia or severe hypokinesia** on echo**, you must consider <u>coumadin</u> to prevent thrombus formation/emboli.**

- **PEARL:** You cannot include a **'lateral' component to an inferior wall MI** if there are only T-wave inversions laterally (must have either ST↑ or Q-waves).

- **PEARL:** For a **posterior component** to the inferior wall MI, look at V1-2 for R>S &/or ST↓ ≥ 2mm. If IWMI + RBBB→can't use this; must do right-sided leads to R/O posterior wall MI.

- **<u>Treatment for Posterior Wall MI and RV Infarction is IVFluids</u> (usually 2 liters NS).**

   ⇒ **Do not give *Nitroprusside*** (Nipride) to patients with RVI: it can markedly reduce the RV and therefore LV preload (primarily due to venodilatation) causing BP to drop dramatically. Efforts must be made to increase preload.

   ⇒ The same goes for **<u>Hypertrophic Cardiomyopathy</u>** by the way. Diuretics, nitrates, and other vasodilators should be avoided since in HCM they will *increase* the obstruction.

PEARL: Remember to look for **T-wave inversions ± ST↓** (and never ST↑) in **<u>Unstable Angina</u>**. *ASA and Heparin* have been proved to decrease mortality in unstable angina.

PEARL: <u>Asymmetric T-waves</u> are 'asymmetric' because they involve ST segment ↑. **Therefore, they usually suggest** acute MI or ischemia

PEARL: **IN DIFFERENTIATING SVT WITH ABERRANCY versus VT,**

One can apply the principal of 'concordance' and 'discordance' fairly easily.

Concordance is where all the main forces in the precordial leads (V1→V6) point in the same direction, i.e. all the R-waves point up or all point down. Concordance suggest *VTach*.

Discordance, on the other hand, is where the main forces in those leads are not in agreement and do not all point in the same direction. Discordance is evidence of *SVT with aberrancy*.

Another trick is to look for the start of the arrythmia and see if you find a **PAC or PVC**. A PAC often precedes SVT with aberrancy, while a PVC often precedes VT.

PEARL: Remember, Digoxin doesn't invert T-waves. **Ischemia** and infarction do.

PEARL: **Digoxin toxicity** can cause a multitude of arrythmias. However, **there are 2 that are the Sine Qua Non of Dig toxicity…**

     1) **SA exit block;**

     2) **PAT with 2:1 block**

And there are 2 arrythmias that digoxin *never* causes…

     1) **Mobitz II;**

     2) **Afib**

PEARL: If you have a **new BBB** with an M.I., besides ASA and angioplasty/lytics, patient needs a **pacemaker**!

PEARL: **Pacemaker syndrome** is sometimes seen in patients with VVI pacemakers who, paradoxically, are short of breath at rest but relieved with exertion. EKG reveals retrograde P-waves.

BUNDLE BRANCH BLOCKS:

LAFB (Left Anterior Fascicular Block) (aka Left Anterior *Hemi*block)
1. QRS between .10-.12 s
2. LAD > - 45°
3. *Small Q in I and L*
4. *Deep S inferiorly*
5. Small R inferiorly

LPFB (Left Posterior Fascicular Block; aka LAHB)
1. QRS between .10-.12 s
2. RAD > +110°
3. *Small Q inferiorly*
4. *Deep S in I and L*
5. Small R in I and L

RBBB—see also next box
1. S wave in I
2. RSR′, T-wave inversion, and ST segment ↓ in V1-V3 (suspect ischemia or infarction is see T-wave inversion or ST↓ laterally)
3. S wave in V5,6
4. *May see ST ↑ inferiorly*.

LBBB-see also next box
1. RSR′, T-wave inversion, and ST segment↓ in I , L, and V4-6 (suspect ischemia or infarction is see T-wave inversion or ST↓ in V1-3)
2. S-waves inferiorly and V1-3
3. *ST↑ in V1-3*

Quickly! Is it a RBBB or LBBB? If the QRS is >0.12s, there is a BBB. You can tell if the BBB is a RBBB or LBBB by finding the location of the RSR′. Very simply, if it is at the right precordium, it is a RBBB. If it is to the left precordium, it is a LBBB.

⇒ Another perhaps even easier way is, once you've determined that the QRS is indeed >.12s and there appears to be a BBB, check the T-wave in V1. If the T-wave is upright, it's a LBBB. If the T-wave is inverted (down), you have a RBBB. A simple **mnemonic** to help you remember this is:
    "When you get RIGHT DOWN to it, it's LEFT UP to you!"

Complete Heart Block (CHB) and AV Dissociation (AVD):
- When the Atrial rate is faster than the Ventricular rate→that's **CHB**.
- When the Ventricular rate is faster than the Atrial rate→that's **AVD**.
- It's really semantics, though, because **BOTH NEED A PACEMAKER.**

AFIB AND CONVERTING TO NSR

- **If atria <5cm & AFib≤ 2 weeks**→may attempt to chemically convert without anticoagulation.
- **If atria < 5cm & Afib present for > 2 weeks**→must give anticoagulation x 3weeks before and after converting
- **If atria > 5cm & AFib present > 2 weeks**→patient is less likely to convert successfully; therefore the goal is to control the ventricular response with, e.g. Digoxin.

CARDIOGENIC SHOCK—4 CAUSES:

1. *RV infarct*→give IV fluids
2. *VSD*→IABP (intra-aortic balloon pump)
3. *Papillary muscle rupture*→→IABP
4. *LV Wipeout* (Massive MI with 2° loss of ≥ 40% of LV)→IABP

INDICATIONS FOR IABP (Intra-Aortic Balloon Pump):

1. Cardiogenic Shock
2. VSD
3. Papillary Muscle Rupture
4. Refractory Unstable Angina
5. VTach presumed 2° to ischemia

VENTRICULAR BIGEMINY (i.e. PVC every other beat)—DDX

1. Hypoxia
2. Thyrotoxicosis
3. Electrolyte imbalance
4. pH ↑or ↑ (alkalosis/acidosis)
5. Ischemia

MAT (Multifocal Atrial Tachycardia)

1. *Heart rate usually >105*
2. *3 different P-wave morphologies*
3. *Seen in COPD classically and commonly*
4. Treatment is Verapamil and, of course, treating the underlying COPD (usually 2° to hypoxia)
5. *Don't give Digoxin (unless MAT progresses to Afib) because you can aggravate the arrhythmia.*

Wandering Atrial Pacemaker can look like MAT in that one can also see at least 3 P-wave morphologies. The key difference is in the rate. WAP rate is usually <95. Essentially, WAP is 'physiologic'; MAT is 'pathologic'.

Approach to the 'Skipped Beat':   First, R/O blocked PAC. You'll identify the **blocked PAC** by noting that the P wave falls right in time/in sync with the other P-waves. Remember the Ashman's phenomenon. Once you've ruled out blocked PAC, you must R/O **Mobitz I** (Type I, 2° Heart Block, or "Wenckebach") by checking for ↑ing PR intervals (and ↓ing R-R intervals) just before the blocked beat.

COMMON CAUSES OF MOBITZ I (WENCKEBACK):

1. Digoxin toxicity
2. IWMI

MALIGNANT EFFUSIONS/TAMPONADE

- **In men→R/O** lung ca.
- **In women → R/O** breast ca.
- Note also, melanoma and lymphoma also metastasize to the pericardium

COMMON CAUSES OF BLOOD PERICARDIAL EFFUSIONS:

- Metastases
- Uremia
- TB

ADVANTAGES OF BETA-BLOCKERS IN CHRONIC CAD

1. Good control of stable angina, particularly exercise-related
2. Anti-HTN
3. Antiarrhythmic effects
4. Possible benefit in preventing sudden death, limiting MI size, or preventing the occurrence of MI should intense ischemia occur
5. Long-acting, reasonably cardioselective, reasonably inexpensive

INTERVENTIONS THAT HAVE BEEN SHOWN TO ↓ MORTALITY AFTER MI:

1. **ASA**
2. **Thrombolytics/angioplasty**
3. **Beta-blockers**→beware in those with severe asthma. Beta-blockers work by decreasing the myocardial wall stress and the cardiac work load. Remember to follow the PR interval (<.24), the HR (>45), the SBP (>100), and check for rales before each dose of IV Beta-blockade. (a 5-5-5mg IV metoprololol at >2 min intervals is commonly used). MI patients should be continued on Beta-blockers, advancing to 50mg PO q6h x1 day, and then to 100mg PO bid indefinitely as tolerated.
4. **ACE Inhibitor 3 days out** (only those with evidence of CHF or low EF% (≤40%) or cardiomegaly should remain on the ACEI)—these work to prevent so-called "remodeling" which can have an ill-effect following an MI.

- While *nitrates* relieve pain, i.e. ↓ morbidity, they *do not ↓ mortality*. Don't get fooled.
- *LV function* is the best prognosticator after MI.
- *Beta-blockers post-MI* have the greatest impact on survival in individuals with compensated CHF c/w those without CHF.

THE DIFFERENCE IN SURVIVAL AFTER M.I. ATTRIBUTABLE TO THESE INTERVENTIONS :

1. ASA→23%↑
2. Lytic therapy→20%↑
3. B-Blocker→ 9%↑
4. ACE Inhibitor 3 days out→7%↑

11. CARDIOLOGY II

Commonly Asked Material ❂...

1. Recognize **Erythromycin** can ↑ digoxin levels as well as anticoagulant levels if used concomitantly; also ↑ risk of rhabodmyolysis when used in conjunction with lovastatin.

2. Usually several questions on **ASD**.

    a) Recognize that it gives a fixed split S2

    b) Biatrial enlargement on EKG

    c) Elevated pulmonary pressure

    d) 2 types: *secundum* (no endocarditis prophylaxis necessary; RAD) and *primum* (prophylaxis necessary; LAD)

3. Recognize the need for **Calcium Gluconate.** Severe hyperkalemia requires emergent treatment directed at minimizing membrane depolarization, shifting K^+ into cells, and promoting K^+ loss. In addition, exogenous K^+ intake and antikaliuretic drugs should be discontinued. Administration of calcium gluconate decreases membrane excitability. The usual dose is 10 mL of a 10% solution infused over 2 to 3 min. The effect begins within minutes but is short-lived (30 to 60 min), and the dose can be repeated if no change in the electrocardiogram is seen after 5 to 10 min.

4. Know the treatment of **Unstable Angina** as opposed to Acute M.I., i.e. ASA, beta-blockers, heparin, etc.

5. Recognize that **thrombolytics** can in fact be used in the elderly, even 80 yo or older, but know the contraindications in general for lytics.

6. Know which **anti-HTN meds** would be potentially dangerous (**increase the block**) in patients with preexisting increased PR/ QRS/ QTc intervals (i.e. already have block), e.g. Calcium Channel Blockers and the IA antiarrythmics, etc.

7. Recognize the patient that would benefit from a **CABG**: *left main disease or 3 vessel disease with LV dysfunction.*

8. Know that **Beta Blockers** have been definitely shown to decrease mortality and recurrence after an M.I.

9. Know that RV infarct and AV block are major complications following **Inferior Wall M.I.**

10. Recognize the **hemodynamics of RV Infarct and Tamponade** (e.g. equalization of pressures in tamponade):

	RA	**PCWP**	**CO**
RVI	↑↑	↓	↓↓
Tamponade	↑↑	↑↑	↓↓

11. Know the clinical manifestations of **tamponade**: hypotension; JVD (and Kussmaul's sign)*; pulsus paradoxus*; electrical alternans. In pulsus paradoxus, the decrease in systolic arterial pressure that normally accompanies the reduction in arterial pulse amplitude during inspiration is accentuated.

In patients with pericardial tamponade, airway obstruction, or superior vena cava obstruction, the decrease in systolic arterial pressure frequently exceeds the normal decrease of 10 mmHg and the peripheral pulse may even disappear completely during inspiration.

12. Usually 1 or 2 questions on **free wall rupture** following acute Anterior Wall M.I.; recognize *EMD* in this setting. The clinical presentation typically is a sudden loss of pulse, blood pressure and consciousness while the electrocardiogram continues to show sinus rhythm (*apparent* electromechanical dissociation). The myocardium continues to contract, but forward flow is not maintained as blood escapes into the pericardium.

13. Know that you can treat **papillary muscle rupture** (with secondary mitral regurg) following acute M.I. with a balloon pump.

14. Know also that an **intraaortic balloon bump (IABP)** can also be used to treat refractory unstable angina; VSD; cardiogenic shock; and VT presumed secondary to ischemia.

15. Recognize **calcific pericarditis** on a CXR.

16. Recognize that severe **dilated (congestive) cardiomyopathy** on lisinopril (or other ACE inhibitor) and diuretics would benefit from addition of digoxin.

17. Know that quinidine, verapamil, thiazides, erythro, & amiodarone can **increase your digoxin level**.

18. Recognize when **nitroprusside** (Nipride) would be indicated (and contraindicated!)

19. Know which types of patients would benefit from an **EPS** (e.g.WPW or recurrent arrythmias following an acute M.I. presumed to be from a single nidus of scar tissue, etc)

20. Usually 2 or 3 questions on **WPW...**
    a. Of course be able to recognize the delta waves on EKG, e.g. in a young man/athlete with
    b. syncope;
    c. ***Procainamide*** for rate control ***when these patients go into Afib or Aflutter***. Digitalis and intravenous verapamil are contraindicated in patients who have WPW syndrome plus AF, since these drugs can shorten the refractory period of the accessory pathway and can increase the ventricular rate, thereby placing the patient at increased risk for VF.
    d. ***Radiofrequency catheter ablation*** of bypass tracts is the treatment of choice in patients with symptomatic arrhythmias.
    e. ***EKG findings*** in WPW syndrome: Short PR interval ; wide QRS complex; and slurring on the upstroke of the QRS produced by early ventricular activation over the bypass tract yielding the delta wave. Inferiorly, delta waves may appear as Q-waves, mimicking myocardial infarction—hence the term "pseudoinfarction" pattern.

21. Know that of all the **Goldman criteria** (re: preoperative), the S3 is the most important risk factor or prognosticator.

22. Complete heart block (third degree heart block and Mobitz II second degree block) as well as some symptomatic bradycardia→**pacemaker**.

23. RBBB + LAHB after acute M.I.→pacemaker.

24. Know the differential of "**Cannon A waves**":
    a) The term implies atria contracting vs. a closed A-V valve
    b) DDx includes: Tricuspid Stenosis; RV Hypertrophy; and Pulm HTN.

25. Know when and why to use **adenosine** (re: can be diagnostic and therapeutic in SVT)

26. Know that we don't use **lidocaine** "prophylactically" anymore peri-MI as it can actually ↑ mortality.

27. Know indications for **cardioversion** in an awake individual→ arrhythmia causing low BP *with symptoms*.

28. Be able to recognize a **Roth spot** (re: the retinal finding from endocarditis/septic emboli).

29. Know who needs (or doesn't need!) **endocarditis prophylaxis**.

30. Usually no congenital heart disease questions, other than ASD and VSD,

31. Recognize the presentation of **Malignant HTN**, especially schistocytes and mental status changes; nitroprusside as drug of choice.

32. **ACE inhibitors** *contraindicated* in **pregnancy**; so is Sulfa (unless she is HIV+ and develops PCP)

33. Recognize a classic case of **cholesterol emboli** post cardiac cath to renal arteries (acute ↑ creatinine; oliguria/anuria) and distal extremities (esp. toes).

34. Recognize that ASA is insufficient for perioperative **DVT prophylaxis** e.g. peri total hip replacement.

35. Know that a **pregnant woman** would use **SQ Heparin** for her anticoagulation, dose-adjusted.

36. Know what to do for a **pulsating abdominal mass**, say 3, 5, and 7 cm (using cutoffs of 4 and 6 cm).

37. Should know how to adjust Heparin in **DVT management** based on PTT, when to start Coumadin (≤ PTT therapeutic but after initiating heparin of course), and when to stop Heparin (INR therapeutic).

38. Changes in **Cardiac Physiology during 3ʳᵈ trimester of Pregnancy**:

    a) ↑: Blood *volume*, Cardiac *Output* (so easier to remember also ↑ stroke *volume* and heart rate)
    b) ↓: SVR (systemic vascular resistance)

CARDIOLOGY NOTES

COMPLICATIONS BY SITE OF MI
- ✪ *Anterior MI*
    1. Ventricular arrythmias
    2. LV aneurysm
    3. Free wall rupture; VSD
    4. Mobitz II
- ✪ *Inferior MI*
    1. Bradycardias, CHB
    2. Papillary muscle dysfunction (common) or rupture (rare)
    3. Associated RV infarction
    4. Mobitz I

ANTICOAGULATION IN NONVALVULAR AFIB: CURRENT RECOMMENDATIONS ✪

	Age <65	Age 65-75	Age >75
Risk factors for CVA	Warfarin	Warfarin	Warfarin
No risk factors	ASA	Warfarin *or* ASA	Warfarin

FACTORS INCREASING THE RISK OF STROKE IN PATIENTS WITH A FIB
Clinical Parameters
1. Increasing age
2. Rheumatic Heart Disease
3. Previous MI
4. HTN
5. H/O previous thromboembolic events

Echocardiographic
1. Global LV Dysfunction
2. Enlarged LA

NYHA (NY Heart Association) Criteria for Assessing Cardiorespiratory Capacity
1. NYHA I—Dyspneic only on severe exertion
2. NYHA II--Dyspneic walking up hills, stairs
3. NYHA III-Dyspneic walking on level ground
4. NYHA IV-Dyspneic at rest

TYPES OF PULSES
1. Alternans—severe left ventricular failure
2. Bisferiens—mixed aortic valve disease
3. Collapsing—AI; patent ductus arteriosus
4. Jerky—IHSS (hypertrophic cardiomyopathy)
5. Paradoxus—tamponade; constrictive pericarditis; asthma
6. Plateau—AS

DDx OF IRREGULARLY IRREGULAR PULSE (i.e. not just Afib!)
1. A Fib, A tach or A flutter with varying block
2. MAT; WAP (wandering atrial pacemaker)
3. PVCs
4. Sinus Arrythmia

THE JUGULAR VENOUS PULSE
1. **Normal**
   a. 'a' wave→right <u>a</u>trial systole
   b. 'v' wave→<u>v</u>enous filling
   c. 'x' descent→atrial rela<u>x</u>ation
   d. 'y' descent→tricuspid opening
2. **Abnormal 'a' wave**
   a. Absent→A Fib
   b. Giant→Tricuspid or Pulmonary stenosis; Pulm HTN
   c. Solitary→Complete Heart Block (CHB)
3. **Cannon waves**
   a. Regular→nodal rhythm
   b. Irregular→CHB; ventricular ectopy
4. **Systolic (ventricular) waves**→tricuspid incompetence
5. **Rapid 'y' descent**→constrictive pericarditis; tricuspid incompetence
6. **Slow/absent 'y' descent**→ tamponade; tricuspid stenosis
7. **Rapid 'x' descent**→ constrictive pericarditis; tamponade
8. **Fixed elevation**→SVC syndrome
9. **Absent Hepatojugular reflux**→IVC obstruction, or Budd Chiari Syndrome

DDX OF A SOFT 1ST HEART SOUND (S1)
1. 1st degree AV block
2. Cardiomyopathy, LVF
3. Large pericardial effusion
4. MR
5. MS with rigid valve

DDX OF LOUD S1
1. Mitral stenosis with mobile valve
2. Sinus tach (e.g. thyrotoxicosis)
3. WPW

TYPES OF SPLIT S2
1. *Fixed split→ASD*
2. Loud A2→systemic HTN
3. Narrow split with loud P2→Pulmonary HTN
4. *Paradoxical (P2<A2)→LBBB*
5. Physiologic—normally A2 is heard before P2, and this widens on inspiration.
6. Single S2 (inaudible A2)→calcific AS
7. Wide split with soft P2→Pulmonary Stenosis
8. Widely split→RBBB

FIXED SPIT S2
1. =ASD
2. Misdiagnoses:
    a) Opening snap (mitral stenosis), simulating P2
    b) Midsystolic click (MVP), simulating A2

DDx of "S3"(*true S3 may be physiologic or 2° to CHF and is due to ventricular volume overload*)
1. Fixed split S2 in ASD
2. MS opening snap
3. MVP with mid-systolic click
    - **_S4, incidentally,_ may be seen in *xclt physical conditioning/HTN/CAD* and is _2°_ _to ↓ ventricular compliance to filling_.**

S3→ *Markedly* diminished LV diastolic function
S4→ *Moderately* diminished LV diastolic function

CHARACTERISTICS OF INNOCENT MURMURS
1. **S** atisfactory EKG and CXR
2. **S** hort duration (half of systole)
3. **S** ingle S2 on exhalation while standing
4. **S** oft, low-pitched
5. **S** upine position best for hearing
6. **S** ystolic ejection murmur

LATE SYSTOLIC MURMURS-DDX
1. Coarctation of aorta
2. Hypertrophic cardiomyopathy
3. MVP
4. Pulmonary arterial stenosis

SYSTOLIC MURMUR FOLLOWING AN MI ✪
1. Misdiagnosis→Dressler's syndrome (pericardial rub seen after transmural infarctions)
2. MR 2° to cardiac incompetence
3. Papillary muscle dysfunction (common) > rupture > rupture of chordae tendinae (uncommon)
4. Ruptured interventricular septum (VSD)→check for harsh murmur palpable thrill

SIGNS INDICATING VALVE MOBILITY IN MS
1. Loud S1
2. Opening snap

SIGNS INDICATIVE OF SEVERE MS

1. Graham-Steel murmur (functional PI) or TI
2. Left atrial enlargement, RVH
3. Length of diastolic murmur
4. Proximity of opening snap to S2
5. RV strain pattern, elevated RV pressures
6. Signs of pulmonary HTN/congestion

SEVERITY OF MS BY ECHO GRADING OF CROSS-SECTIONAL VALVE AREA

1. Valve area (in square cms) >2.5 →asymptomatic
2. Valve area 1.5-2.5→symptoms on exertion only
3. Valve area .5-1.5→symptoms at rest
4. Valve area < .5→"severe"

- *Remember too that patients with MS who have a slow heart rate tend to do better.*

DDX OF THE MS DIASTOLIC MURMUR

1. *Austin-Flint murmur* (mitral flow murmur of severe **AI**)
2. *Graham-Steel murmur* (severe **MS** + Pulm HTN→this PI murmur)
3. Flow murmurs in volume overload
   a) Severe MR
   b) VSD, PDA
   c) Renal failure
4. LA myxoma –think of this too in patients who syncopize while recumbant or have postional pre-syncope/syncope.

ARE THEY SYSTOLIC OR DIASTOLIC?!

Remember, "(h)**AR**d **AS**s **MR**s. **MS**d", in other words…
   AR→diastolic
   AS→systolic
   MR→systolic
   MS→diastolic

LEFT ATRIAL MYXOMA

1. Loud or soft S1; *'tumor plop'*
2. Pansystolic murmur
3. Symptoms are postural, e.g. syncope
4. Mass seen on echo
5. DDx on echo…
   a) LA thrombus
   b) Large MV vegetation
   c) Thick or redundant MV leaflets

CLINICAL CORRELATES OF MVP ✪
1. ASD
2. IHSS
3. Ischemic or rheumatic heart disease
4. Marfan's syndrome; Ehlers-Danlos syndrome
5. PAN
6. PCO
7. WPW

INDICATIONS FOR VALVE REPLACEMENT IN AI
1. Symptoms
2. Declining exercise tolerance on stress testing
3. ↑ heart size on CXR
4. Development of LV strain pattern
5. LV end-systolic diameter>55mm in an asymp patient as seen by echo
6. ↓ in EF% on echo or MUGA

CAUSES OF AI
1. Bicuspid AV
2. HTN
3. Valvulitis
   a) Rheumatic
   b) Infective
   c) Rheumatoid arthritis
4. Aortitis
   a) Syphilis
   b) Ankylosing Spondylitis

SYMPTOMS AS PROGNOSTICATORS IN AORTIC STENOSIS ✪
1. <u>A</u>ngina→death within 3-5years (if untreated)
2. <u>S</u>yncope→death within 2 years
3. Dyspnea→death within 1 year
4. Overt cardiac failure→death within 6mo.

> **Pearl:** *The later the peak* of the systolic murmur→the <u>worse</u> the AS.
> Similarly, *the loss of S2* connotes a <u>worse</u> AS

> **Pearl:** In AS, valve areas ≤ 0.75 cm^2 are considered "critical".

SOME INDICATIONS FOR *PERMANENT* PACING
1. Alternating RBBB and LBBB
2. Complete Heart Block
3. Drug-resistant tachyarrythmias
4. Intermittent Mobitz II A-V block
5. Symptomatic bradyarrythmias, e.g. SSS (Sick Sinus Syndrome)
6. Symptomatic patient with bi- or tri-fascicular block and prolonged H-V interval

INDICATIONS FOR *TRANSVENOUS* PACING IN ANTERIOR MI
1. 2° or 3° AVB
2. Alternating RBBB and LBBB
3. New LBBB with pre-existing 1°AVB
4. New RBBB with pre-existing 1° AVB/LAHB/LPHB

ACC/AHA Guidelines for Implantation of ICDs (Implantable Cardioverter-Defibrillator)
1. Cardiac arrest due to VF or VT not due to a transient or reversible cause
2. Spontaneous sustained VT
3. Syncope of undetermined origin with clinically relevant, hemodynamically significant sustained VT or VF induced at EPS when drug therapy is ineffective, not tolerated, or not preferred
4. Non-sustained VT with CAD, prior MI, LV dysfunction, and inducible VF or sustained VT at EPS that is not suppressible by a class I antiarrythmic.

✪ **PEARL:** Following MI (esp in those with non-sustained VT), **EPS** (to study inducibility of VT) and checking for **late potentials** are excellent ***risk stratifiers for sudden death*** if they are negative. That is, they are valuable based on their ***negative predictive value***.

ADVERSE PROGNOSTIC FINDINGS ON EXERCISE EKG STRESS TESTS ✪
1. ↑ in complex ventricular ectopy (along with ST-segment shifts)
2. Exercised-induced typical angina
3. Low peak heart rate (e.g. <120 bpm without pacemaker)
4. Low workload (e.g., <6.5 METs or 5-6min on Bruce protocol)
5. Marked ST segment depression (eg. >2mm)
6. Prolonged ST-segment depression (e.g. >6min) after exercise
7. SBP ↓ (e.g. >10mm Hg from baseline) or flat response (peak<130mm Hg)
8. ST-segment depression in multiple leads
9. ST-segment elevation without abnormal Q wave

CARDIAC SYNDROME X: MAIN CLINICAL FEATURES
♦ Exercise-induced chest pain, so + EST
♦ Atypical features of chest pain (e.g. prolonged episodes, poor response to sublingual nitrates)
♦ Negative stress echo
♦ Normal coronary angiogram
♦ Abnormal pain perception in many patients
♦ Microvascular angina in some patients
♦ Antianginals ineffective in ~ 50% of patients
♦ Good prognosis regarding survival
♦ More common in women with estrogen deficiency than those without deficiency.
♦ Still somewhat ill-defined

FEATURES OF VALVULAR HEMOLYSIS
1. Signs of gross (para)valvular regurgitation
2. Normochromic normocytic anemia
3. Schistocytes on peripheral smear
4. ↓Haptoglobin with negative Coombs' test

INDICATIONS FOR TISSUE (PORCINE) VALVES
1. Any patient with absolute contraindication to anticoagulation
2. Elderly patient in NSR with normal size left atrium requiring MVR
3. Elderly patient requiring AVR
4. Young woman desiring pregnancy

♦ *Remember*, the key difference between tissue and prosthetic valves is that tissue valves don't require anticoagulation. While prosthetic valves require anticoagulation, these valves last much longer.

VERAPAMIL—ABSOLUTE CONTRAINDICATIONS:
1. Digoxin toxicity (re: dig ↑s the levels of quinidine or verapamil by 50%, and vice versa)
2. High degree AVB
3. Hypotension, heart failure
4. Sick Sinus Syndrome
5. Simultaneous IV Beta-blockers
6. WPW

CONTRAINDICATIONS TO DIGOXIN THERAPY
1. AVB
2. WPW; MAT
3. Prior to elective cardioversion
4. Constrictive pericarditis; acute myocarditis
5. Hypertrophic CMP in NSR

INDICATIONS FOR CHECKING SERUM DIGOXIN LEVEL
1. Suspected toxicity
2. Refractory Afib
3. Appearance of new arrythmias
4. Change in renal function
5. Initiation of new treatment, esp. quinidine/amiodarone/spironolactone/verapamil.

ARRYTHMIAS IN DIGOXIN TOXICITY
1. Most any bradycardia or block
2. PAT with 2:1 block (classic)
3. Sino-atrial exit block

• *Never see*: Afib or Mobitz II from Digoxin toxicity.

CAUSES OF A FIB ✪ → Remember → "**PIRATES**":

P E, pericarditis
I schemia
R heumatic Heart Disease
A trial Myxoma
T hyrotoxicity
E thanol
S tenosis (mitral)

and...HTN (#1 cause)

INDICATIONS FOR EPS IN TACHYARRYTHMIAS
1. Wide-complex tachycardias unable to be distinguished from VT
2. Recurrent VT
3. Recurrent SVT with...
   a) Hemodynamic compromise
   b) Syncope
   c) WPW on resting EKG

DDX OF WIDE-COMPLEX TACHYCARDIA
1. SVT with aberrant conduction (see discordance)
2. VT (see concordance)
3. WPW with anterograde conduction (look for delta waves)

ASSOCIATIONS OF WPW
1. Male sex; familial
2. MVP
3. Thyrotoxicosis

> ✪ **Arrhythmias seen in WPW: PAT is by far the most common; Afib is #2. These account for the large majority. Procainamide is excellent at treating WPW with 2° Afib.**

EKG MANIFESTATIONS OF SSS
1. **Prolonged episodes of sinus bradycardia**
2. Profound sinus arrythmia with symptoms of tissue hypoperfusion
3. Periods of sinus arrest (>3s)
4. Junctional escape rhythms
5. **'Tachy-brady' syndrome (backround bradycardia punctuated by paroxysmal bursts of Afib or flutter)**
6. Chronic Afib (end-stage sinus node dysfunction)

NEW GUIDELINES FOR HEART FAILURE TREATMENT ✪

- **High dosages of ACE I**
- **Digoxin**
  - ⇒ Patients who *should not* receive digoxin include those with advanced AV block or those with asymptomatic heart failure. In general, too, dig should be avoided in the acute phase after MI.
  - ⇒ Digoxin *may not* be effective in patients who have normal LV systolic function
  - ⇒ The benefits of dig are greatest in patients with severe CHF, an enlarged heart, and an S3.
- **Diuretics** (*esp. spironolactone*—but beware of ↑K with concurrent use of ACE inhibitor
- **Beta-blockers** (e.g. Bisoprostol, Carvedilol, Metoprolol—all characterized in major clinical trials)
  - ⇒ *Now considered standard therapy*
  - ⇒ Nearly all patients with heart failure are considered candidates for β-blockers
  - ⇒ Most patients with diabetes can safely use β-blockers
  - ⇒ PVD is not considered a contraindication to the use of β-blockers
  - ⇒ *Initiate β-blocker in CHF only after patient is stable on an ACEI, digoxin, and a diuretic.*
  - ⇒ Also recommended, of course, for use post-MI

> ✪ *Remember*: 1) The treatment for *dilated, i.e. 'congestive' CMP* is *also* ACE inhibitor/dig/diuretics; 2) When a patient presents in *CHF with a normal EF%*, one should R/O CAD and valvular heart disease; and 3) When you see increasing azotemia with diuretics yet no improvement in symptoms of CHF, this suggest low EF% / forward failure, which necessitates *positive inotropy treatment* (e.g. dobutamine or milrinone).

DIAGNOSES TO CONSIDER IN REFRACTORY CHF

1. PE
2. Silent MI
3. Silent valvular stenosis
4. Anemia
5. Cardiac tamponade; constrictive pericarditis
6. High-ouput failure in elderly (thyrotoxicosis; Paget's dz)
7. LV aneurysm
8. Myocarditis
9. Overvigorous hydration
10. Thiamine deficiency

CXR CORRELATION WITH PULMONARY CAPILLARY WEDGE PRESSURES

1. Dilated upper lobe veins→PCWP=15 mmHg
2. Kerley B lines→20mmHg
3. Pulmonary edema→25mmHg

INDICATIONS FOR RIGHT HEART CATHETERIZATION
1. Uncertainty about the patient's volume status
2. Comorbid conditions, including ongoing ischemia, sepsis, renal insufficiency, or severe lung disease.
3. Lack of response to empiric therapy.

FEATURES DISTINGUISHING RESTRICTIVE CMP FROM CONSTRICTIVE PERICARDITIS
1. No pulsus paradox
2. No Kussmaul's sign (re: Kussmaul's sign also seen in RVI; rare in tamponade)
3. Low-pitched S3
4. Cardiomegaly/LVH
5. No pericardial thickening/effusion
6. Certain hemodynamics
   a) LVEDP>RVEDP
   b) RVSP>60mmHg

FEATURES DISTINGUISHING HCM FROM AS ✪ (essentially they react opposite on all maneuvers below)
1. +FH-- premature sudden death
2. Apex beat--double impulse
3. Murmur is late systolic (not ejection); inaudible in carotids
4. Maneuvers (Incidentally, the MR murmur of MVP behaves exactly as per HCM below)
   a) HCM **murmur ↑** by valsalva/standing/nitrates (all **with decreased left ventricular volume which in turn ↑the outflow obstruction**)
   b) HCM **murmur ↓** by squatting/isometric exercises (by **increasing LV volume**)

> ✪ Echocardiographic findings characteristic of IHSS: '**SAM ASH**'→ "**S**ystolic **A**nterior **M**otion of the anterior MV leaflet with **A**symmetric **S**eptal **H**ypertrophy"

EMD (Electrical-Mechanical Dissociation)—DDx ✪ :   "**HH PP TT**" :

Cause	*Usual Intervention*
H ypotension	Bolus IVF
H ypoxia	Hyperventilate
P E	"
P H↓ (i.e. acidosis)	"
T ension pneumothorax	Chest tube
T amponade	Pericardiocentesis

Biochemical Markers of Cardiac Injury:

Marker	Cardiac Speficicity	Initial Rise	Duration of Elevation
Cardiac Troponin I	++++	4-6 h	4-7 d
Cardiac Troponin T	++++	3-4 h	10-14 d
CK-MB	++	3-4 h	1-1 ½ d

KEY CAUSES OF UNILATERAL LOWER EXTREMITY SWELLING

Acute Swelling (<72 h)
DVT
Popliteal cyst
Rupture of medial head of the gastoc
Bacterial cellulitis
E. nodosum

Chronic Swelling (>72 h)
Lymphedema
Chronic venous insufficiency
Reflex sympathetic dystrophy
Malignancy

THROMBOLYTICS ✪

If you see true **angina (t<12h from time of onset) + ST↑ (≥2 leads)** or if you see **angina + new BBB→thrombolytics** are justified in the ER setting (assuming no contraindications to thrombolytics) .

Absolute contraindications include: 1) prior intracranial bleed or CNS tumor; 2) recent prolonged CPR; 3) active internal bleeding; 4) CVA or head trauma within the previous 6 months; and 5) use of Streptokinase for the second time in a year (since patient builds up antibodies to it and tends to react poorly the second time if used so soon after.

Relative contraindications include: 1)GIB within 1 month; 2) surgery or trauma in the past 2 weeks; 3) pregnancy; and 4) BP >200/110.

Mechanisms of More Common Lytic Agents:
1. **TPA**→high affinity for fibrin: clot specificity
2. **Streptokinase**→Combines with circulating plasminogen to form a proteolytic complex
3. **APSAC**→Same as streptokinase since it is metabolized to SK after injection.

✪ Following AWMI, approximately 1/3 patients will develop *mural thrombi*.

HYPERTENSION:

- Know the *JNC* VI (or most recent) clinical definitions for adult **BPs**:

Category	Systolic		Diastolic
Optimal	<120	and	<80
Normal	<130	and	<85
High-normal	130s	or	85-89
HTN			
Stage 1	140s-150s	or	90s
Stage 2	160s-170s	or	100-109
Stage 3	>=180	or	>=110

- The *diagnosis of HTN* requires *at least* 2 formal measurements on different days.

  - *Isolated systolic HTN* affects mainly the elderly.

  - In HTN patients, *LVH* is a strong negative prognosticator for sudden death and MI.

  - **Certain drugs** can cause HTN; classic ones include:
    1. *OCPs*—induce Na+ retention
    2. *NSAIDs* also induce Na+ retention, but by blocking formation of vasodilating, natriuretic prostaglandins.

HTN AND CO-MORBIDITY ☉

Condition	Anti-HTN Drug class or agent
DM with proteinuria	ACE inhibitors
CHF	ACE inhibitors, diuretics (esp. spironolactone), carvedilol, losartan
Isolated systolic HTN in elderly patients	Diuretics, long-acting CCBs
M.I.	Beta-blockers, ACE inhibitors (if CHF or↓EF%)
Angina	B-blockers, CCBs
AFib/Atach	B-blockers, CCBs
NIDDM without proteinuria	Diuretics
Dislipidemia	Alpha-blockers
Essential tremors	Beta-blockers (non-cardioselective)
Hyperthyroidism	Beta-blockers
Migraine	Beta-blockers (non-cardioselective), CCBs
Osteoporosis	Thiazides
Preoperative HTN	Beta-blockers
Renal insufficiency	ACE Inhibitors

CARVEDILOL
1. Non-selective beta-blocker
2. *Also* an alpha-blocker
3. Peripheral vasodilator effect
4. Most importantly, carvedilol is used in severe CHF, helping to ↑ the EF%;
5. *↓morbidity AND mortality*

CONSERVATIVE RECOMMENDATIONS (prior to or in combination with medication)
1. ↓ Weight;
2. ↓ Fat intake
3. ↓Smoking
4. ↓Alcohol to < 2oz/day
5. ↓ Na+
6. ↑Regular exercise

MERIDIA AND XENICAL: A Summary of the New Weight Loss Meds		
Med	**Mechanism of action**	**Side effects**
Sibutramine (Meridia®)	Reuptake inhibitor of serotonin, NE, and dopamine	↑BP, tachycardia, H/A, insomnia constipation, dry mouth
Orlistat (Xenical®)	Reversible lipase inhibitor	Fecal incontinence, oily spotting, flatulence, vitamin malabsorption

VERAPAMIL

1. Should be avoided in SSS (sick sinus syndrome) as well as 2nd or 3rd degree blocks.
2. Avoid using with CHF when EF<40%
3. **↑ risk of digoxin toxicity**
4. Most common side effect=constipation

FMD (FIBROMUSCULAR DYSPLASIA)

1. Classic string-of-beads appearance on renal angiography
2. #1 cause of renovascular HTN in younger persons, esp women< 25

ATHEROMATOUS RENOVASCULAR DISEASE

1. #1 cause of renovascular HTN in elderly
2. Frequently bilateral
3. Bruit heard 50% of the time
4. Onset after 50 yo
5. ↓K+ due to 2° aldosteronism
6. *Remember, the sudden ↓ in renal function with the use of an ACE I should make you think of Bilateral RAS (renal artery stenosis).*
7. Remember too with RAS, captopril scan is the screening method of choice, as it is safe in pts with renal insufficiency or history of allergy to contrast media. Doppler Duplex U/S may also be considered but is very "operator dependent", meaning the results are only as good as the tech performing the study.

ATHEROEMBOLIC RENAL DISEASE ✪

1. History is key→e.g. Occurrence *after angiography or aortic surgery*
2. *Livedo reticularis and peripheral emboli* (manifest as gangrene toes, e.g.)
3. Rapid decline in renal function
4. Sudden worsening of HTN

RENAL PARENCHYMAL DISEASE

1. #1 cause of 2° HTN
2. HTN (in turn) and DM are the biggest causes of renal parenchymal disease.
3. Remember, other than peripheral cortical scarring (seen with HTN renal dz), *renal size* (using U/S) is probably the easiest way to differentiate CRF secondary to HTN (kidneys smaller) vs. Diabetes (an infiltrative dz, therefore, kidneys larger)

PRIMARY HYPERALDOSTERONISM

1. Excess aldo(from unilateral adenoma or B/L hyperplasia) *leads to* HTN and ↓ K+ and ↓ renin
2. Suspected in pts with spontaneous *↓K+* or precipated by usual dose diuretic therapy.
3. Clinical: muscle *weakness;* cramps; H/A; palpitations.
4. *EKG* changes: ↑ ST; inverted Ts; U waves.
5. Dx: after a 3-day high salt diet, measure Na+, K+, creatinine, and aldo in a 24 h urine.
   - a *24 h urine aldo*>12 ng (if urine Na+>200meq) is diagnostic.
6. Tx: adenoma→*surgery*;
   hyperplasia (if no mass seen on adrenal CT) →*spironolactone*

PHEOCHROMOCYTOMA

1. Extra-adrenal tumors are only norepi-producing, whereas adrenal pheos may be epi- or norepi-producing tumors.
2. *"Rule of 10's"*:
   10% of pheos are extraadrenal
   10% are malignant
   10% are familial
   10% are bilateral (since familial tumors tend to be bilateral)
3. *Common presentation*: H/As; sweating; palpitations; HTN *and* orthostatic hypotension.
4. *Screen* with 24 h urine for metanephrines (VMA) and catecholamines (Epi, Norepi).
5. *Next* step: Abdom CT to locate the tumor (for surgery)
6. *Preop*: administer alpha blockers followed by beta-blockers.

COARCTATION OF THE AORTA

1. May go undetected beyond childhood
2. Key → *Upper extremities* HTN, esp. relative to lower extremitiess (low BP/cold feet)
   → Also may see *rib notching* on CXR.

HTN IN PREGNANCY ✪

1. BP ↓s in early pregnancy
2. **Preeclampsia** → *triad* of **HTN, edema, and proteinuria** developing **after the 20th week**.
   - Can see ↑ **uric acid**, which you would *not* see with chronic HTN in pregnancy.
3. **Eclampsia** → preeclampsia *plus* **convulsions**.
   - *Warning signs*→H/A, blurry vision, epigastric pain, hyperreflexia, or cerebral symptoms.
   - **Magnesium** sulfate for impending eclampsia; *calcium gluconate* for *mag* toxicity!

4. Tx for HTN in pregnancy
    - **Methyldopa** is recommended initial therapy
    - **ACE inhibitors contraindicated.**

MALIGNANT HTN ✪

1. Sudden severe ↑ in BP associated with acute injury to target organs.
2. Retinal hemorrhages, exudates, papilledema frequently noted
3. *HTN encephalopathy*→papilledema, H/A, confusion, GI distress, seizures.
4. *Schistocytes* (fragmented rbcs) seen on blood smear.
5. HTN Emergency--*Nitroprusside* is the drug of choice.

    - May result in cyanotoxicity if thiocyanate levels are not checked Q48h
    - Na+Nitrate and Hydroxycobalamin (Methylene Blue) used to treat toxicity.
    - Side effects of Nitroprusside: N/V, agitation, flushing, fasciculations and tremor.

HYPERTENSIVE CRISES

EMERGENCIES *(DBP>115 <u>with</u> evidence of end-organ dysfunction or damage)*[1]
1. Accelerated-malignant HTN (most cases)
2. Acute GN
3. Acute LVF with pulmonary edema
4. Acute or impending MI
5. Dissecting aortic aneurysm
6. Drug-induced acute HTN
7. Eclampsia
8. HTN with acute CVA
9. HTN encephalopathy
10. Intracranial hemorrhage
11. Unstable angina

[1] BP should be lowered *gradually* over 2-3 hours to SBP 140-160 and DBP 90-110. To avoid cerebral hypoperfusion, the BP should not be lowered by > 25% of the MAP (mean arterial pressure). Except for ecclampsia, *nitruprusside* can be used for almost hypertensive emergencies.

URGENCIES *(DBP>115 <u>without</u> end-organ dysfunction/damage; gradually reduce BP over 24-48h)*
1. Accelerated-malignant HTN (some cases)
2. HTN with optic disk edema
3. Progressive target organ complications
4. Severe perioperative HTN
5. Upper levels of stage 3 HTN

CLINICAL FEATURES OF ACCELERATED-MALIGNANT HTN

BP→usually > 130-140 diastolic
Cardiac→CHF
Fundoscopy→hemorrhages, exudates, papilledema
General→malaise, weakness, fatigue, weight loss as a result of salt and water loss
GI→N/V
Hematologic→ anemia due to chronic renal disease or microangiopathic hemolysis
Neurologic→H/A, somnolence, altered MS, visual symptoms, focal deficits, seizures, coma
Renal→azotemia, proteinuria, hematuria

PREDOMINANT RENOVASCULAR DISEASE by AGE:
1. Fibromuscular dysplasia→age usually < 30yo
2. Atherosclerosis→age usually >60yo

HIGH AND LOW RENIN STATES AS RELATED TO HTN

	No HTN	HTN
↑Renin	Addison's dz Hemorrhage Liver dz Pregnancy Drugs* Bartter's syndrome	Malignant HTN Essential HTN (in 15%) Renovascular HTN ESRD Reninoma
↓Renin	Elderly Drugs**	Essential HTN (85%) Conn's syndrome Cushing's syndrome CAH Corticosteroids

* Diuretics, estrogens, vasodilators
** Beta-blockers, clonidine, methyldopa.

SEE NEXT PAGE FOR HYPERLIPIDEMIAS

	Problem	Plasma	Presentations	Treatment
HYPERLIPIDEMIAS ✪				
Type I	Deficiency of lipoprotein lipase	↑ TG ↑ chylomicrons Creamy layer of supernatant after overnight incubation	*Eruptive* xanthomas Pancreatitis	Fat free diet Medium chain TG Fat-soluble vitamin
Type IIA	Deficiency of LDL receptors or overproduction of Apo B	↑LDL ↑TC	*Tendon* xanthomas Premature atherosclerosis and CAD	HMG CoA reductase inhibitor + Bile acid binding resins
Type IIB	↓ LDL and VLDL receptors	↑LDL ↑VLDL	Mixed	HMG CoA reductase inhibitor or Nicotinic acid
Type III	Abnormal Apolipoprotein E	↑LDL ↑VLDL	*Palmar & tuberous* xanthomas; Premature atherosclerosis and CAD DM; hypothyroidism	HMG CoA reductase inhibitor or Nicotinic acid
Type IV	Overproduction of Apo B and VLDL	↑ VLDL	Premature atherosclerosis and CAD	Gemfibrozil or Nicotinic acid
Type V	Mixed I + IV	↑Chylomicrons ↑VLDL Creamy supernatant after overnight incubation	*Eruptive* xanthomas Pancreatitis CAD	Gemfibrozil and/o Nicotinic acid + Low fat diet

12. Pulmonary and Critical Care Medicine

TUBERCULOSIS

TREATMENT OF PULMONARY TB

1. Suspect Drug Resistance→ R.I.P.E. until sensitivities return
2. Then, if INH-Sensitive → R.I.P. x 2 mo→ R.I. x 4 more months.
3. If INH-Resistant,→ R.E. ± P x 18 months (or 12 months after sputum culture negative, whichever is longer)

MDR-TB (MULTI-DRUG RESISTANT TB)
1. Implies resistance to at least 2 drugs, usually INH and Rifampin
2. Risk factors include
    a. Recent immigration from Latin America or Asia
    b. Living in area of ↑ resistance (≥ 4%)
    c. Previous Rx without Rifampin
    d. Previous incomplete treatment
    e. Exposure to known MDR-TB
3. Associated with a high mortality
4. Requires treatment with ***at least*** 3 drugs from among the following, <u>e.g.</u>

R ifampin +	***OR***	**S** treptomycin or Capreomycin or Kanamycin +
I NH +		**A** mikacin +
P ZA +		**F** loroquinolone
E thambutol		

Generally, you want to…
♦ **Give ≥ 3 drugs until culture becomes negative, including any first-line agent to which the patient is partially sensitive, ≥ 1 injectable agent (streptomycin, capreomycin, or kanamycin), and, possibly, a quinolone.**
{Typical MDR-TB regimen: R.I.P., oflaxacin, cycloserine, and capreomycin}
♦ **Then give 2-drug regimen for ≥ 12 months after culture-negative.**

5. Note, may consider Rifabutin, instead of Rifampin, as ~30% of Rifampin-resistant strains are Rifabutin-sensitive.

TWO-STAGE TST (TB SKIN TEST) ✪
1. Use in **individuals who are tested regularly** for TB, e.g. nursing home residents.
2. *The idea* → Because the immune response may wane with time/age, elderly patients may require a second "booster" test dose 1 week later to see if the first neg test was a false negative. The second dose should "wake-up" the immune system and help to identify a h/o TB exposure. Remember this is the appropriate testing in nursing home patients.

3. Also, if the first stage is +, but < 10mm→repeat in 1 week, and if then≥ 10mm, you can safely say this is *not a recent conversion* to directly diagnose recent converters. **In other words, recent converters will not have a boostered response.**

Note: **Steroids** are absolutely contraindicated in **TB** *unless* the patient is receiving maximal anti-TB therapy and there is acute hypoadrenalism (Addison's) due to TB infiltration/ablation of the adrenals. Other controversial exceptions include: TB Pericarditis; Acute Miliary TB with septic shock; and TB meningitis.

POTENTIALLY MISLEADING CLINICAL PRESENTATIONS OF TB

Presentation	Misdiagnosis
Night sweats, hilar lymphadenopathy	Lymphoma
H/A, Nausea, Meningismus, CSF Leukocytosis with Negative Gram Stain	Viral Meningitis
Bloodstained ascites	Abdominal malignancy

TOXICITY OF ANTI-TB MEDICATIONS:

1. **INH** (Isoniazid)
   a) Hepatitis
   b) SLE
   c) Pyridoxine deficiency (rare)→neuropathy
   d) Potentiation of phenytoin, coumadin
2. **Rifampin**
   Daily Administration
      a) Antagonism of OCPs, warfarin, steroids, digoxin, and short-acting sulfonylureas
      b) Asymp ↑ of AST, ALT
   Intermittent Administration
      a) Hepatitis
      b) Orange-red discoloration to urine, tears
      c) Flu-like illness
      d) Hemolysis, ITP, DVT, azotemia
3. **Streptomycin**
   a) Hypersensitivity reactions—rash, malaise, ↑eos
   b) Vestibular damage (esp if renal impairment)
   c) Teratogenicity
4. **Ethambutol**—optic neuritis, esp in renal impairment
5. **PZA** (Pyrazinamide)—hepatotoxicity in 10%

WHO GETS INH AGAIN? ✪

	AGE	
Category	**<35 yo**	**≥35 yo**
With risk factor [1]	**Yes, if PPD ≥10mm (or >5 if HIV+, recent contact, CXR with old-not active-TB)**	**Yes, if PPD ≥10mm (or >5 if HIV+, recent contact, CXR with old-not active-TB)**
No risk factor/high incidence group [2]	**Yes, if PPD≥ 10**	**No INH**
No risk factor/low incidence group	**Yes, if PPD≥15**	**No INH**

[1] **Risk factors include:** HIV, IVDA, recent contact with infected person, recent PPD converters, old TB on CXR, and patients with certain medical conditions (silicosis, CRF, DM, immunosuppression, hematologic malignancy, CXR shows old TB, and S/P gastrectomy or jejunoileal bypass).

[2] **High incidence group's include:** foreign-born persons, medically underserved, low income populations, and residents of long-term care facilities.

- **N.B.** A PPD≥ 10mm is considered + for MTB exposure even in patients who have been vaccinated using **_BCG_** in their country, secondary to ↑prevalence population.

INFLUENZA
1. Type A most common
2. Those ≥65yo have by far the highest mortality
3. Strep and Staph can secondarily infect
4. **Amantadine** is only effective vs. Type A and can shorten the course of disease in influenza only if given **within 48 hours** of symptom onset (Amantadine as _TREATMENT_)
5. Amantadine + Vaccine confers ± 95% protection (Amantadine as _PROPHYLAXIS_)
6. Amantadine toxicity = restlessness, insomnia, dizziness, renal
7. The flu vaccine **may in fact be given along with Pneumovax**
8. The following **risk groups** should receive annual vaccine:
    a) ≥65
    b) > or < 65 with chronic medical problems, such as cardiopulmonary disorders and DM
    c) Health care personal
    d) Nursing home residents and residents of other long-term care facilities, as well as their staff
    e) House-hold members of high-risk groups
    f) Healthy pregnant women who will be in their 2nd or 3rd trimesters during the flu season.
    g) HIV and immunocompromised
    h) Anyone who wishes to reduce the likelihood of becoming ill with influenza

9. Be ready to recognize the value of the newer agents, **Relenza** (zanamivir)—for inhalation-- and **Tamiflu** (oseltamivir)—supplied as capsules--, both **neuraminidase inhibitors**, in uncomplicated acute illness due to influenza virus if symptomatic **for ≤ 2 days**.

DDX of WHEEZING + EOSINOPHILIA
1. **ABPA**
2. **Churg-Strauss**
3. **PAN**
4. **Strongyloides**

- **Löeffler's syndrome** is not included in this list since, while there are transient pulmonary infiltrates and peripheral blood eosinophilia, *there is no wheezing*.

WEGENER'S GRANULOMATOSIS
1. **Pulmonary-renal syndrome (others include** Goodpasture's; Churg-Strauss; SLE; Cryoglobulinemic vasculitis; Leukocytoclastic vasculitis, i.e. small vessel vasculitis)
2. **c-ANCA** (Remember, "Yes, WE c-AN")
3. Pulmonary manifestations include hemorrhage and thick-walled, centrally-**cavitating nodules**
4. Renal manifestation is **Focal Segmental** GN
5. The mnemonic "**ELKS**" summarizes the organs affected:

> **E** NT ('saddle nose' deformity; nasal discharge; paranasal sinusalgia)
> **L** ung
> **K** idney (involvement usually follows E/L/S of ELKS)
> **S** kin

- *Think Wegener's if see* **triad of sinusitis + hemoptysis + large cavitary nodules on CXR**

GOODPASTURE'S SYNDROME ✪
1. *Hemoptysis* is usually always the initial symptom
2. *Pulmonary* involvement typically *precedes* renal involvement; **P**-ANCA
3. Serum ELISA technique can detect *anti-basement membrane antibody*
4. *Plasmapheresis* is an important adjunct to immunosuppression in reducing this auto-Ab

> **Generally, lung biopsy is preferable in diagnosing Wegener's, while a renal biopsy is preferable in diagnosing Goodpasture's.**

BORDETELLA PERTUSSIS
1. Responsible for **whooping** cough
2. Should R/O in cases of **prolonged bronchitis** in older children and adults
3. May cause ↑↑Lymphocytes
4. Treatment with **Erythromycin**

CHLAMYDIA PSITTACOSIS
1. Asymptomatic avian carriers→poultry workers, e.g. cleaning out bird cages
2. F/C, H/A, dry cough, stiff neck; TCN is treatment.

LEGIONNAIRE'S DISEASE ✪
1. Clinical: weakness, malaise, **high fever**, **cough**, and **diarrhea**, relative bradycardia, **bilateral patchy infiltrates**
2. Labs: **↓Na, ↓ Phos,** ↑ WBC, **↑ LFTs**
3. **Diagnosis:**
   a) **Urine Antigen-1**
   b) √ Ab with **IFA** (Indirect fluorescent Ab) test; ≥ 1:256 or a 4-fold ↑ is pos.
4. Treatment: Erythro ± Rifampin; Fluoroquinolone; or Azithromax

MISCELLANEOUS PEARLS FOR THE BOARDS ✪
- In **massive hemoptysis**, the cause of death is usually asphyxiation, not exsanguination (bleeding out

- **Hypertrophic Pulmonary Osteoarthropathy** is generally caused by *adeno ca and large cell* ca of the lung. It can be seen on bone scan.

- **Horner's syndrome** consists of the triad of ptosis, meiosis, and anhydrosis. It is 2° to superior sulcus tumors (Pancoast tumors) which is usually caused by SVC syndrome or Squamous Cell Ca of the lung.

- **HRCT** (High Resolution CT) is the investigational tool of choice for diagnosing **bronchiectasis**.

- *Bronchial artery embolotherapy* can lead to *spinal artery embolism* which in turn can present with **neurologic deficits, since the spinal artery is a branch of the bronchial artery.**

- An ↑ **serum ACE level** does not establish the dx of sarcoidosis, since it is non-specific and may be elevated in a variety of other conditions such as mycoses and hyperparathyroidism.

- Know that a patient can tolerate a pneumonectomy if her **preop FEV1 (as well as most indices) > 50% of predicted**.

- Remember, in **emphysema**, air trapping leads to hyperinflation, **a ↓ in elastic recoil, and an ↑ in compliance**. Remember from way back? → compliance & elasticity are *inversely proportional*. You might want to think of an old rubberband to understand this concept: the older it gets, the more you can stretch it (more compliance), but it won't shoot as far (less recoil).

COMMON CAUSES OF A CHRONIC COUGH (> 3 wk) ✪
1. **Asthma**
2. **Chronic bronchitis**
3. **GERD**
4. **Post-nasal drip**
5. **ACE Inhibitor**

COMMON CAUSES OF COPD→ "ABCDE" ✪

A sthma—*reversible* airway obstruction
B ronchitis
C ystic Fibrosis
D ilatation of the bronchi (Bronchiectasis)—*irreversible* →look for "train-tracking" on the CXR
E mphysema

- In general, *bronchiectasis* is seen in the *lower lung fields*. Important <u>exceptions</u> include:
    a) Cystic Fibrosis
    b) ABPA
    c) Chronic Mycoses

CYSTIC FIBROSIS ✪

1. + Family History (more common among caucasians)
2. <u>**Sweat Chloride ≥ 70**</u>

3. *Common Complications and Clinical Correlates:*
    a) **Pseudomonal** infection common
    b) **Aspergillus** (ABPA in 10% of Cfers)
    c) **Candida** Albicans
    d) Asthma
    e) **Pancreatic insufficiency**
    f) **Azospermia**
    g) **Infertility (nearly all men and women with CF)**
    h) **Sinusitis**
    i) Purulent sputum
    j) COPD in 90% of adult survivors; **bronchiectasis**
    k) **Hemoptysis** (71%)
    l) Nasal polyps (48%)
    m) Anorexia, weight loss, clubbing

KARTAGENER'S SYNDROME ('Immotile Cilia Syndrome')

1. Half of these patients have situs inversus (i.e. dextrocardia)
2. Sinusitis is common
3. Males are commonly infertile*

- Note: The infertility in Kartagener's syndrome is 2° to **immotility** of the sperm, whereas in CF, it is 2° to **azospermia** (reflecting obliteration of the vas deferens)

HEMOPTYSIS—MOST COMMON CAUSES

1. **B** ronchiectasis; bronchitis
2. **L** ung carcinoma
3. **T** B

OBSTRUCTIVE SLEEP APNEA—CLINICAL FEATURES ✪

1. **Snoring**
2. **AM Headaches**
3. **Feeling poorly rested on awakening**
4. **Daytime drowsiness**
5. **Systemic / Pulmonary HTN**
6. **Ventricular arrythmias** (2° to prolonged periods of apnea at night)
7. Peripheral edema 2° to **Pulm HTN**/cor pulmonale
8. Obstructive sleep apnea **2° to obesity**, the disorder is referred to as **Pickwickian** Syndrome
9. $\downarrow pO2$
10. $\uparrow pCO2$
11. **Polycythemia** 2° to $\downarrow pO2$
12. RVF→LVF in late stages
13. **Nasal CPAP** an important tool in treatment

IDIOPATHIC PULMONARY FIBROSIS (IPF)

1. PFTs show a **restrictive** pattern with $\downarrow$DLCO
2. Any end-stage diffuse lung disease can **mimic** IPF;
    a) BOOP (Bronchiolitis Obliterans with Organizing Pneumonia)
    b) DAD (Diffuse Alveolar Disease)
    c) LIP (Lymphocytic Interstitial Pneumonitis)
    d) etc.
3. BAL (Bronchoalveolar lavage) can be useful in distinguishing IPF from sarcoidosis
    a) Neutrophils predominate in IPF; whereas
    b) Lymphocytes predominate in sarcoidosis.
4. Commonly see **hypoxemia exacerbated by exercise** (similar to PCP)
5. **Lung biopsy** is important in this disease, since the causes are multiple
6. **Honeycombing** on CXR, if seen, is significant, since it signifies **advanced** disease.
7. Prognosis is poor without **lung transplantation**.

BOOP (Bronchiolitis Obliterans with Organizing Pneumonia)

1. Pathology→Seen when bronchiolitis (inflammation and fibrosis of the small airways) spreads to adjacent parenchymal tissue.
2. Etiologies →RA; viral infections; toxic inhalations.
3. CXR→ parenchymal infiltates
4. PFTs→ restrictive defect

SARCOIDOSIS ✪

1. A **systemic disease** of unknown etiology which causes **non-caseating granulomas** throughout the body.
2. Presence of non-caseating granulomas is **_not_ diagnostic** as they can be seen in other diseases, which often also produce hilar lymphadenopathy!
3. Think of this disease if presented with a young black women (W>M, B>F) in her 20's-30's with bilateral hilar LN + E. nodosum.

4. **Staging**/Progression:

Stage I	Hilar *lymphadenopathy*
Stage II	I + pulmonary *parenchymal* disease
Stage III	Pulmonary parenchymal disease *without* hilar LN (*tricky!*)
Stage IV	Pulmonary *Fibrosis with bullae*

5. **False-negative PPD** (2° to suppressed T lymphocyte function)
6. Remember, **serum ACE** levels are non-specific and are **corroborative** *only*.
7. Other labs frequently seen in sarcoidosis:
   a) ↑ vitamin D
   b) Hypercalciuria
8. Know these important **INDICATIONS FOR STEROIDS** in **SARCOIDOSIS**:
   a) Ocular involvement
   b) Cardiac involvement
   c) Neuro involvement
   d) Progressive pulmonary disease
   e) Hypercalcemia
   f) Hypercalciuria with renal insufficiency
   g) Disfiguring cutaneous manifestations (e.g. Lupus Pernio—violacious nodules occurring over the nose and malar regions)

Pulmonary **I**nfiltrates with **E**osinophilia (**PIE**). Here's your PIE (DDx of pulm infiltrates and ↑serum e

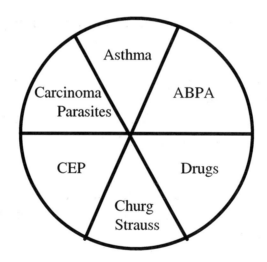

- About <u>10%</u> of <u>asthmatics</u> bear the triad of <u>bronchospasm + ASA sensitivity + nasal polyps</u>.
- Nitrofurantoin can cause fever/cough/pulmonary infiltrates/↑eos.

THE DIFFUSE INTERSTITIAL LUNG DISEASES...

- **Smokers** predisposes to 2 DLDs→ PEG (Pulmonary Eosinophilic Granuloma) and PAP (Pulmonary Alveolar Proteinosis)
- The other name for PEG is Histiocytosis X (might remember **"PEG is His X"**), because of th atypical histiocytes that are found in the tissue.
- ↓DLCO

ILDs THAT CAN GIVE SPONTANEOUS PNEUMOTHORAX
1. **PEG**

2. **LAM** (Lymphangiomyomatosis) (*see next*)

3. Cystic Fibrosis

LAM
1. **Women** of childbearing age
2. Recurrent spontaneous **pneumothorax**
3. **Hemoptysis**
4. **COPD** picture on PFTs
5. Hyperinflation with reticulonodular infiltrates.

ILDs ASSOCIATED WITH HILAR/MEDIASTINAL ADENOPATHY
1. Lymphoma

2. Lymphagitic carcinomatosis

3. Sarcoidosis

ILDs ASSOCIATED WITH A COMBINED OBSTRUCTIVE AND RESTRICTIVE DEFICIT:
1. LAM

2. PEG

3. Sarcoidosis

ASBESTOSIS:

1. **Pleural thickening (esp. apical) ± pleural plaques** best appreciated at the diaphragmatic border. Remember, though, sarcoid and TB also show pleural thickening.

2. Fibrosis usually predominates in the **lower** lung fields (as opposed to silicosis)

3. Due to the resulting fibrosis, PFTs reveal a *restrictive* pattern.

4. Mesothelioma usually follows asbestos exposure by an average of 40years.

5. Another long-term complication of asbestosis is **bronchogenic ca; smoking is markedly synergistic** in this regard. ✪

6. Unlike bronchogenic ca, when **smoking** is added to asbestos exposure, there is **no** additional ↑ risk of developing **mesothelioma.** ✪

SILICOSIS ✪

1. Associated with sandblasting, mining professions.
2. **No ↑ risk of lung ca**
3. **"Eggshell" calcifications** of hilar LNs (a term also used in sarcoidosis)
4. + RF and +ANA are common
5. **If you see fever** with silicosis (± weight loss)→ R/O Silicotuberculosis and **√ a PPD**, as their is a significantly ↑ risk of developing TB in silicosis.

HYPERSENSITIVITY PNEUMONITIS ✪

1. Caused by **fungal** precipitans (thermophilic actinomycetes)
2. Serum precipitins are almost always + for this fungus
3. ↑ Immunoglobulins, except Ig E
4. **+ RF** seen in most cases
5. Clinical presentation: **Fever/Chills/Sweats/Dry cough/ Dyspnea**
6. These symptoms resolve faily rapidly (18-24 hours), and recur on reexposure to the antigens.
7. PFTs are **restrictive**
8. **No wheezing; no eosinophilia**

EXERCISE-INDUCED ASTHMA (EIA)

◆ Patients may complain of wheezing, cough, chest tightness, fatigue, or SOB during or after exercise.
◆ Of course, a resting physical exam may be completely normal.
◆ Dx usually supported when preexercise inhalation of a short-acting β-agonist causes symptom resolution.
◆ *Nonpharmacologic approaches* to EIA as well as advice to patients should include a pre-exercise warm-up, exercising in warm, humid air, and exercising in short bursts.
◆ Short-acting β-agonists are **1st-line drug therapy** for these patients.
◆ Cromolyn and nedocromil are considered **2nd-line therapy** and are effective in 70-85% of patients. They work by inhibiting mast cell degranulation and *should be taken 10-45 min prior to exercise*. Their duration is 1-2 h. They may be used alone or in conjunction with a β-agonist.
◆ Long-acting β-agonists, like salmeterol, may also help, although effects may wane over time.
◆ Leukotriene inhibitors also appear to be beneficial in a 75% of patients in a recent study.

PPH (Primary Pulmonary HTN)

1. 2° to hyperreactivity of the pulmonary vasculature
2. F>M incidence
3. Clinical presentation
   a) **Exertional dyspnea/syncope/presyncope 2° to**...
   b) Pulmonary HTN, which causes 2° cor pulmonale
   c) CXR: Cardiomegaly with prominent pulmonary artery and "pruning" of the pulmonary vessels
   d) ↑ Pulmonary pressures seen on right heart cath
4. Calcium channel blockers, like nifedipine have been successfully used in treatment.

DRUG-INDUCED LUNG DISEASE

DRUG	PULMONARY TOXICITY
Nitrofurantoin/phenytoin/hydralazine	SLE-like picture with pleural effusions (50%) and pulmonary infiltrates (30%); hydralazine→pleurisy.
Narcotics	ARDS; Non-cardiogenic Pulmonary Edema; Granulomas (e.g talc); pneumonia; Bronchiectasis; Endocarditis
'Crack' cocaine	Diffuse alveolar hemorrhage; BO ± OP; hypersensitivity pneumonitis
Busulfan/Bleo*/BCNU*	All can lead to pulmonary <u>fibrosis</u> (Remember to "<u>B.tough</u>") Bleo may also cause a pneumonitis.
Methotrexate	Hypereosinophilia; Hilar LN; pleural effusion
Steroids may predispose to	Nocardia; Mycoses (esp Aspergillus, Candida, Crypto) and may exacerbate TB
ASA overdose	Respiratory Alkalosis (following an anion gap metabolic acidosis)
Prolonged O2 at high FIO2	ARDS
Amiodarone*	Diffuse infiltrates (remember, patients on this amiodarone should have their *PFTs, TFTs, and LFTs* closely monitored.
Penicillamine	BOOP; SLE
Methylsergide	Fibrosis

==

* THE PULMONARY INJURY WITH THESE IS <u>DOSE-RELATED.</u>

- Remember, **<u>High Altitude Pulmonary Edema</u>** occurs among high-altitude natives on returning to altitude after being at sea level.several weeks.

SOLITARY PULMONARY NODULE ✪

1. Large majority are benign; remember the key always is _serial films_; an SPN that shows no growth over 6-9 months is usually benign.

<table>
<tr><td colspan="2">ETIOLOGIES OF SOLITARY
PULMONARY NODULES</td></tr>
<tr><td>Malignant nodules</td><td>40%</td></tr>
<tr><td>Bronchogenic carcinoma</td><td>33%</td></tr>
<tr><td>Other 1° malignancies</td><td>2%</td></tr>
<tr><td>Solitary metastasis</td><td>5%</td></tr>
<tr><td>Benign nodules</td><td>60%</td></tr>
<tr><td>Infectious granulomas</td><td>50%</td></tr>
<tr><td>Benign tumors</td><td>5%</td></tr>
<tr><td>Other</td><td>5%</td></tr>
</table>

2. **_Benign_** SPNs are usually **< 2.5-3cm** in diameter
3. **_Malignant_** SPNs which tend to be **> 3cm**
4. Dx: For more proximal SPNs→can usually do a wedge biopsy. More distal SPNs usually require either a CT-guided or Fluoroscopy-guided transthoracic needle biopsy.
5. The following clinical features are quite useful in **_differentiating_** benign and malignant SPNs:

	More Likely Benign	**More Likely Malignant**
Age	Age <35	Age > 35
Gender	Female	Male
Smoker?	No	Yes
Size	<2.5-3 cm	>2.5-3 cm
Margins	Smooth margins	Irregular margins/spiculated edges
Calcification	Central/popcorn/ laminated calcification	Eccentric calcification
Growth (on CXR)	No	Yes
Satellite lesions	Yes	No
CT scan +C	<20 Hounsfield units	> 20 H.U. enhancement
PET	No uptake (with fluorodeoxyglucose)	↑ uptake

DIAGNOSES VALUE OF GROSS SPUTUM EXAM

1. 'Anchovy sauce'→ Amebic abscess
2. Black→coalworker's pneumoconiosis with progressive, severe fibrosis
3. Clear, watery, copious→Alveolar cell ca
4. Frank blood with simultaneous mucopurulent sputum→TB
5. Pink, frothy→CHF
6. Purulent, malodorous→ Lung abscess; bronchiectasis
7. Rubbery brown plugs→ ABPA
8. Rusty, mucoid→Pneumococcal pneumonia

DDx of ↑A-a (Alveolar-arterial) Gradient→Remember, "VSD" ✪

1. V/Q mismatching, e.g.
   a. PE
   b. Airway obstruction
2. Shunt
   a. Intracardiac (e.g. **VSD!**)
   b. Intrapulmonary (ARDS, CHF)
3. Diffusion defect, e.g.
   a. IPF
   b. Emphysema

INTERPRETING PFT'S "Quick & Dirty" ✪

1. **First**, check out the **FLOWS** (e.g. FEVs): If ↓, then patient usually has **obstructive** disease
2. **Next**, look at the **VOLUMES** (e.g. FVC): If ↓, then patient usually has **restrictive** disease
3. **Then**, look at the **DLCO**: If ↓, patient usually has either emphysema, PPH (Primary Pulmonary HTN, or IPF (Idiopathic Pulmonary Fibrosis)
4. **Finally**, if all the above are normal: Consider a **methacholine challenge to R/O asthma**

✪ Remember also, **FEF 25-75** is one of the best measures of **small airway disease.**

✪ To diagnose **reversible** obstructive lung disease (e.g. asthma), the following parameters should ↑ **in response to bronchodilators: FEV1 or FVC ≥15% or FEF 25-75 ≥ 50%.**

✪ A sudden ↓ **in the FEV 1 by ≥ 20% is an indication for hospitalization**.

• In patients with COPD, *exercise tolerance correlates more with FEV 1*, in general, than with their pO2.

✪ **Home O2 is indicated** for patients with pO2 <55 or O2 sat% <88.

DDx of ↑ DLCO ☻
1. Alveolar hemorrhage
   a) Mitral Stenosis
   b) Goodpasture's syndrome
   c) Trauma, etc.
2. Polycythemia
3. Acute asthma

DDx of ↓ DLCO (↓ *surface area available for gas exchange*) ☻
1. **IPF**
2. **Emphysema**
3. **PE**
4. **PPH (1° Pulm HTN)**
5. Sarcoidosis
6. Anemia

- **Pancreatitis** predominantly lateralizes to the **left** when it causes pleural effusions.
- **CHF and cirrhosis** tend to give **right**-sided pleural effusions.

CRITERIA FOR AN EXUDATIVE PLEURAL EFFUSION (≥1 OF THE FOLLOWING)
1. Pleural fluid/serum **total protein ratio > .5**
2. "   "   "   **LDH** ratio **> .6**
3. Pleural fluid LDH > 2/3 of the upper limit of normal serum LDH (traditionally)
4. Pleural fluid pH > 7.3

SPECIALIZED TESTS FOR DETECTING CAUSES OF PLEURAL EFFUSION	
Test	**Diagnosis**
TG> 110 mg/dl	Chylothorax
Amylase >200 U/dl	Esophageal perf; malignancy; pancreatic dz; ruptured ectopic pregnancy
RF ≥ 1:320 and ≥ serum titre	Rheumatoid effusion
ANA ≥1:160 and ≥ serum titre	Lupus pleuritis
CEA >10ng/dl	Malignancy
Adenosine deaminase >43U/L	TB pleuritis

COMMON DDX OF TRANSUDATIVE PLEURAL EFFUSIONS
1. ↓Albumin
2. CHF (#1 cause)/cirrhosis (ascites)/nephrosis
3. Constrictive pericarditis; SVC syndrome
4. Iatrogenic
5. PE

COMMON DDX OF <u>EXUDATIVE</u> PLEURAL EFFUSIONS: *(mostly 1°pulmonary processes)*
1. Pulmonary / pleural malignancy
2. Pneumonia; Empyema; other pulmonary infections
3. PE (yes, here too!)

> ✪ **If there is any suspicion of TB or malignancy, a pleural biopsy should be taken (in addition to thoracentesis). However, pleural fluid cytology is more sensitive for malignancy.**

COMMON CAUSES OF PLEURAL EFFUSIONS WITH ↓ PLEURAL FLUID GLUCOSE ✪
1. Empyema
2. Esophageal rupture (esp with ↓pH and ↑amylase)
3. RA (esp. if also find ↓pH and ↑LDH)
4. TB (don't forget pleural biopsy if suspect)

AGE-RELATED CHANGES IN PULMONARY FUNCTION ✪
1. ↓FEV
2. ↓ VC
3. ↑FRC (Functional Residual Capacity) and ↑ in RV
4. ↓ in pO2
5. There is no ↑ in pCO2 with aging

<u>IMPORTANT DIAGNOSTIC LINKS</u>   **<u>DIAGNOSIS TO LOOK FOR</u>**

• Recurrent sinusitis + infertile young adult male	Kartagener's syndrome
• Chronic productive cough + DM in young adult	Cystic Fibrosis
• Productive cough on most days ≥ 3mo ≥ 2 consecutive years	Chronic bronchitis
• Obstructive lung dz + lower lung bullae + hepatic inflammation	Alpha-1 antitrypsin deficiency

ALPHA-1 ANTITRYPSIN DEFICIENCY
1. An inherited disorder
2. May lead to liver disease, *emphysema* or both in some individuals
3. It has been shown that liver transplantation restores normal levels of this enzyme, so appears to play a critical role in this disease.
4. The emphysema is more severe at the <u>*lung bases*</u>

HRCT ESPECIALLY USEFUL IN:
1. Bronchiectasis
2. LAM
3. Lung mets
4. PEG
5. Patient with diffuse interstitial infiltrates of unclear cause

MODERN APPROACH TO THE DIAGNOSIS OF PULMONARY EMBOLUS:

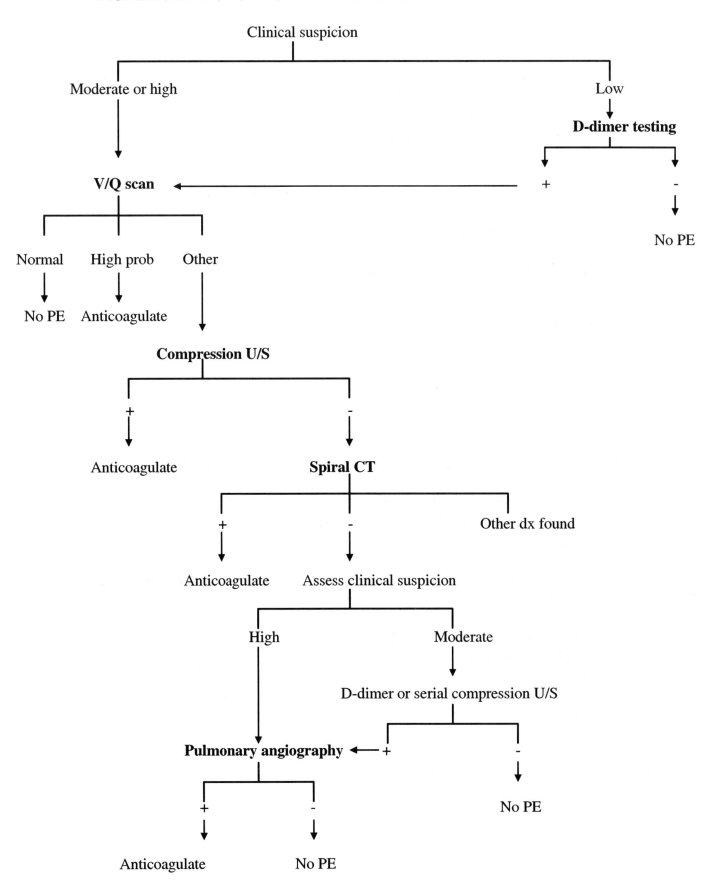

> ✪ *Remember*, in V/Q scanning, a normal scan essentially rules out PE, and an angiogram should follow an indeterminate scan if your clinical suspicion is high.

TESTING FOR PE WITH A D-DIMER ASSAY:

> ✪ *A D-dimer assay can help rule out PE in patients with nondiagnostic lung scans or a low pretest probability of disease:*

- For those patients with a **low pretest probability** of disease and a normal D-dimer result, the D-dimer assay has been shown to yield a <u>negative predictive value of 99%</u>.
- For those with a **nondiagnostic lung scan** and a normal assay, the D-dimer assay has been shown to have a <u>negative predictive value of 97%</u>.

> • Transbronchial needle aspirations are often done during bronchoscopy in the diagnosis of mediastinal lymphadenopathy. This procedure is commonly known by pulmonologists as "Wang needle aspiration".

MRI IS PARTICULARLY USEFUL IN DIAGNOSING THE FOLLOWING:
1. Tumor involving the A-P window
2. Tumor invading the chest wall
3. Superior sulcus tumors
4. Small perihilar tumors

PULMONARY INVOLVEMENT IN RA
1. Caplan syndrome (pneumoconiosis + rheumatoid nodules in the lungs)
2. Crycoaretenoid joints affected→upper airway obstruction may be seen.
3. Interstitial fibrosis
4. Obliterative bronchiolitis
5. Pleural effusions (re: low glucose)
6. Restrictive picture to PFTs and/or ↓DLCO
7. Subpleural rheumatoid nodules (usually only seen with high titres RF or when additional features are present)

THEOPHYLLINE dose should be monitored especially closely when used in:
(all of the following slow the rate of elimination of theo ✪)
1. CHF; COPD
2. Obesity
3. OCPs
4. Severe liver disease
5. Simultaneous use of cimetidine, erythromycin, fluoroquinolones (e.g. cipro), digoxin, verapamil, propranolol, allopurinol, and OCPs.

> ✪ <u>*Smoking*</u>*, on the other hand, causes theophylline to be more rapidly cleared; hence theophylline dose should be adjusted upwards as appropriate.*

THEOPHYLLINE TOXICITY—PRIMARILY 3 SYSTEMS…
1. **Neuro**→tremor/seizures; insomnia
2. **Cardiac**→arrythmias
3. **GI**→N/V

POOR PROGNOSTICATORS IN COPD
1. ↓FEV 1
2. Cor Pulmonale
3. Poor ABG findings
4. Tachycardia

A COMPARISON OF THE MAIN SMOKING-RELATED COPDs:

Emphysema	vs	**Chronic Bronchitis**
'Pink Puffers'		'Blue Bloaters'
Dyspnea		Coughing
Hyperventilation ("pink puffer")		No hyperventilation
No cyanosis		Cyanosis ("blue") Right heart failure→edema ("bloater")

SILO-FILLER DISEASE
1. 2° to inhalation of **nitrous oxide**
2. Causes **non-cardiogenic pulmonary edema**
3. May see symptoms in 2 patterns, early (immediately after exposure) and weeks later.

CHRONIC EOSINOPHILIC PNEUMONIA (CEP) ✪
1. Diffuse interstitial infiltrates in the peripheral lung fields. When bilateral, this is referred to as the "**photonegative**" of pulmonary edema.

2. **Asthma and BOOP** are common associations

3. **Eosinophilia** in the blood and lung tissue
4. May also see ↑ platelets, ↑↑ESR, and an Fe def anemia
5. **Unlike PEG, it responds well to steroids**

DRUGS WHICH CAUSE NON-CARDIOGENIC PULMONARY EDEMA
1. Opiates (heroine; morphine; methadone)
2. ASA
3. Propoxyphene (Darvon®)

ARDS ✪

1. Remember, the **wedge (PCWP) is normal** (as opposed to CHF); compliance is decreased
2. **Hypoxemia** is the major clinical manifestation
3. **Sepsis is the #1 cause** (trauma, burns, pancreatitis are just some of the many other causes)
4. **PEEP** is an important resource to use because:
   a. It prevents alveolar collapse
   b. It plays an important role in recruiting collapsed alveolar units
   c. It allows you to dial down the FIO2 that might otherwise cause further damage that actually resemble ARDS. This usually occurs at levels ≥ 60% FIO2 for >24 hours.
   d. Beware, though, as PEEP can cause a drop in the cardiac output.
5. Carries a high mortality

VENTILATORS ✪

Ventilator SETTINGS:

♦ **To affect the pH or pCO2, you adjust the RATE and/or TIDAL VOLUME. The rate is usually altered first**

♦ **To affect the pO2 or sat%, the FIO2 and/or PEEP are usually adjusted, usually the FIO2 first.**

[Recall that a normal pH=7.40; a normal pCO2=40; a normal pO2 is about 100.]

♦ The only other ventilator setting is the MODE. The most common modes are IMV, SIMV, CPAP, and Assist Control. It is important to know how each of these modes work.

✪ **Intermittent Mandatory Ventilation (IMV).** In this mode, the machine provides a preset number of breaths each minute. The patient can breath on his/her own, but the machine may cycle on during a patient breath. As the rate is dialed down, the patient assumes more of the work of breathing. This can lead to patients "bucking the vent", often alleviated by changing to AC mode (below).

✪ **Synchronized IMV (SIMV).** As per IMV above, except that the machine senses the patients own breaths, allowing her to finish her breaths before cycling on.

✪ **Continuous Positive Airway Pressure (CPAP).** The machine provides no breaths, but does provide air at a preset FIO2 with a constant airway pressureThe patient does all of the ventilation in this mode, but remains connected to the ventilator primarily for monitoring purposes. It is useful as a test before extubation. IMV is also used as a weaning or exercise mode. So is **"T-piece"**, which is often likened to *breathing through a large straw* to exercise the respiratory muscles before extubation. Patients usually rest at night on Assist Control mode (*see next*).

✪ **Assist Control (AC).** *This is the usual preferred initial mode.* The patient initiates a breath and the machine cycles on to deliver the preset tidal volume. Essentially the machine senses the negative inspiratory pressure exerted by the patient and **"assists"** the patient by helping with the remainder of the inspiratory effort. If the patient fails to make a breathing effort altogether, the machine has a **"back-up rate"** or set number of breaths that is delivered anyways.

ADJUSTING THE SETTINGS: GENERAL RULES OF THUMB...

- **When the pO2 is high**, lower the FIO2. Use the **Rule of 7's** to guide your adjustment in FIO2: For every 1% decrease in FIO2, the pO2 will drop by 7. So, for example, if the pO2 is 310 on 80% FIO2, take 310-100 (goal)=210, which is the amount of decrease we will need to make in the pO2. Dividing 210 by 7, we see we need to lower the FIO2 by 30. So 80%-30% leaves 50%, which is where we should order the new FIO2 in order to bring down the pO2 to 100.
- If the pO2 is   high and your FIO2 is already low, then the PEEP can be lowered (usually in increments of 2 with follow-up blood gases). Because of oxygen toxicity, patients with a high pO2 should have their FIO2 lowered first, then the PEEP.

- *Conversely*, **for low pO2s**, one should similarly first adjust the FIO2 up before adjusting the PEEP. Let's briefly reiterate several important points about PEEP:
    PEEP is an important resource to use <u>because</u>:
    - a. It prevents alveolar collapse
    - b. It plays an important role in recruiting collapsed alveolar units
    - c. It allows you to dial down the FIO2 that might otherwise cause further damage that actually resemble ARDS. This usually occurs at levels $\geq 60\%$ FIO2 for >24 hours.
    - d. Beware, though, as PEEP can cause a drop in the cardiac output.

- **When the pCO2 is high**, this typically indicates hypoventilation, so, assuming our tidal volume is set at 10-15cc/kg, simply dial up the rate first.

- *Conversely*, **when the pCO2 is low**, this usually indicates hyperventilation (for whatever reason) and either the rate should be lowered, or, if it is noted the patient's spontaneous breaths (not machine-delivered breaths) are tachypneic, then sedation or even paralysis with further evaluation may be necessary.

COMPLIANCE
<u>2 Types of compliance</u>: static and dynamic

$$\textbf{Static Compliance} = \frac{\text{Tidal Volume}}{(\textit{Plateau} \text{ pressure-PEEP})}$$

$$\textbf{Dynamic Compliance} = \frac{\text{Tidal Volume}}{(\textit{Peak} \text{ pressure-PEEP})}$$

RECOGNIZING COMMON VENTILATOR PROBLEMS:

Problem	$\rightarrow$	Usual Answer
High peak pressure		Mucus plugging
Low pressure (peak) alarm		Cuff leak/cuff rupture
High peak and plateau pressures		Pneumothorax, CHF common
Low compliance		ARDS

WEANING

Weaning Criteria:
Before starting to wean the patient from the machine, these parameters should be met:
1. FIO2 <40%
2. PEEP<5
3. PaO2>60
4. Patient alert and stable

The patient must have adequate ventilation on their own; therefore, the:

5. NIF (negative inspiratory force) must be ≥ -25 (more negative); and
6. TV (tidal volume)>400 in a normal sized adult;
7. Vital Capacity > 10cc/kg

Important Weaning Modes
1. T-piece
2. CPAP
3. SIMV

Choice of Weaning Mode
⇒ *T-piece and CPAP* weaning are good options for patients who have undergone mechanical ventilation for short periods and therefore do not require much in the way of respiratory muscle reconditioning. *SIMV* is better for patients who have been intubated for prolonged periods and therefore require gradual respiratory muscle reconditioning.

Doing the Actual Wean
- ✪ **T-piece weaning** involves brief spontaneous breathing exercises or trials with supplemental oxygen. Trials are usually initiated for 5 min/h and are typically followed by a 1-h rest interval (on AC mode, or "resting mode"). T-piece trials are gradually increased in 5- to 10-min increments until the patient demonstrates that s/he can remain off the vent for several hours at a time. Extubation can then be tried.
- ✪ **CPAP weaning** is similar to weaning on the T-piece except that trials of spontaneous breathing are done while the patient is physically on the ventilator in CPAP mode. This is usually done *with pressure support* (PS), which one can liken to another PS, "power steering", since pressure support serves to "drive" the breath in (pardon the pun), making it easier for the patient to pull the entire breath.
- ✪ **SIMV weaning** entails gradually lowering the mandatory backupor machine rate in increments of 2-4 breaths per minute while monitoring the patient's blood gases and respiratory rates. Respiratory rates > 25 usually indicate respiratory muscle fatigue and the need to combine such trials with periods of rest. Exercise periods are progressively increased until the patient can tolerate this mode all the way down to 4 breaths per minute. T-piece or CPAP trials can then be attempted before considering extubation.

13. ENDOCRINOLOGY

Hypogonadism

- Semen analysis almost always abnormal
- ↓ SHBG (Serum Hormone Binding Globulin); ↓ serum Testosterone is not specific for hypogonadism.

- Primary gonadal failure→see ↑ LH, FSH
- Secondary gonadal failure ("hypogonado**trop**ism")→ see ↓ LH, FSH; one should therefore also evaluate the rest of the pituitary functions.
    - These pairs should be analyzed together…
    a)   FSH level↔semen analysis
    b)   LH level ↔Testosterone level

- If patient presents with delayed puberty + *anosmia/hyposmia* (abnormal development of olfactory lobes)→*Kallmann's Syndrome*

Klinefelter's Syndrome

- 47 XXY
- *Clinical*
    1. Small, firm testes
    2. Azospermia; infertility
    3. ↓ testosterone
    4. ↑LH, FSH
    5. Gynecomastia (incidentally, unilateral gynecomastia should make one think of carcinoma)
    6. Eunuchoidism
    7. Positive buccal smear (for karyotyping)
- Treated with Testosterone supplements—remember to delay supplementation as long as possible to allow for closure of the epiphyses to allow appropriate growth.

Male infertility
Common causes
    1. Abnormal sperm count/quality
    2. Ductal obstruction (e.g. 2° to varicocele—90% are left-sided)
    3. Ejaculatory disorders

Azospermia—physician must differentiate #1 from #2; FSH levels and sometimes testicular biopsy (ouch!) can settle.

Impotence (1° vs. 2°)

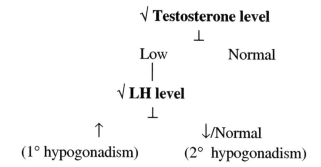

√ **Testosterone level**

⊥

Low   Normal

|

√ **LH level**

⊥

↑   ↓/Normal

(1° hypogonadism)   (2° hypogonadism)

TFM (Testicular Feminization) ✪

1. Genetic males affected with ambiguous genitalia (thus aka "*Male Pseudohermaphroditism*")
2. Lack the enzyme *5 alpha-reductase* for *peripheral conversion of testosterone to its active form, DHT* (dihydrotestosterone), in the tissues.
3. At adolescence, normal breast and female 2° sex characteristics seen; however, no pubic hair and no menarche
4. Managed with *gonadectomy after puberty completed*

Turner's Syndrome
- Female phenotype
- 45XO
- **Clinical**—may see…

    1. Short stature

    2. Webbed neck

    3. Low-set ears

    4. Small jaw (micrognathia)

    5. Short metacarpals/metatarsals

    6. Epicanthal folds

    7. Shield-like chest

    8. ↑ carrying angle at the elbows

    9. Coarctation + Aortic Stenosis

    10. Amenorrhea—in fact this is the #1 cause of 1° amenorrhea

- Turner mosaics may have none of these stigmata and may present with either 1° or 2° amenorrhea.

Amenorrhea ✪

- Remember that the #1 cause of amenorrhea and ↑PRL is *pregnancy*!
- *Ovarian disorders* are common causes of 2° amenorrhea; *PCO* (Polycystic Ovary Syndrome is the most common of these).

    ◊ The diagnosis is often made by recognizing an *obese, hirsute* patient with complaints of abnormal menses. An ↑LH/FSH ratio (>2:1) is common in this disorder. ↑PRL in ½-1/3 of these pts.

- *"Postpill" amenorrhea* accounts for 30% of 2° amenorrhea; it occurs in 2% of women taking BCPs; 30% of *those* have *hyperprolactinemia*; remember, psychotropic drugs (**phenothiazines), haloperidol, and metoclopramide** can ↑ PRL levels→2° amenorrhea.

- HyperPRL accounts for 25-40% of all 2° amenorrhea;

- *1° hypothyroidism* is also a common cause

- If adult female sex characteristics are present and neg βHCG→R/O *structural causes* of amenorrhea as well as *TFM*.

- If patient is sexually infantile, R/O 1° amenorrhea, checking *hormone levels*.

Hirsutism ✪

- Diagnosis--The idea is to figure out if *the androgens are coming from the <u>ovary</u>* or from the <u>*adrenals*</u> (congenital adrenal hyperplasia; adrenal tumor)

- *DHEAS levels:*   **<u>DHEAS is an adrenal androgen</u>**
  <7 ng/dl→ excludes adrenal tumor or CAH→→then check Testost.
  >7 ng/dl→DDx includes **adrenal tumor or CAH**

- *Testosterone:*   >200→→Suspect **ovarian tumor**.
  <200→→PCO

- ↑ T + ↑ DHEAS → adrenal cause
- ↑ T only → ovarian cause

- *Other hyperandrogenic signs* that may be appreciated...
    1. Acne
    2. Abnormal menses
    3. Clitorimegaly
    4. Masculinization
    5. Defeminization

ALGORTHMIC APPROACH TO WORKUP...

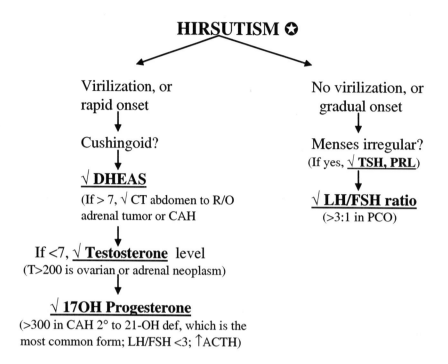

HIRSUTISM ✪

Virilization, or rapid onset

Cushingoid?

√ DHEAS

(If > 7, √ CT abdomen to R/O adrenal tumor or CAH

If <7, √ **Testosterone** level
(T>200 is ovarian or adrenal neoplasm)

√ 17OH Progesterone
(>300 in CAH 2° to 21-OH def, which is the most common form; LH/FSH <3; ↑ACTH)

No virilization, or gradual onset

Menses irregular?
(If yes, √ **TSH, PRL**)

√ LH/FSH ratio
(>3:1 in PCO)

THE RELATIONSHIP BETWEEN THE CORTISOL AND ANDROGEN SYNTHESIS PATHWAYS: <u>GONADAL & ADRENAL</u> SOURCES OF ANDROGENS ✪:

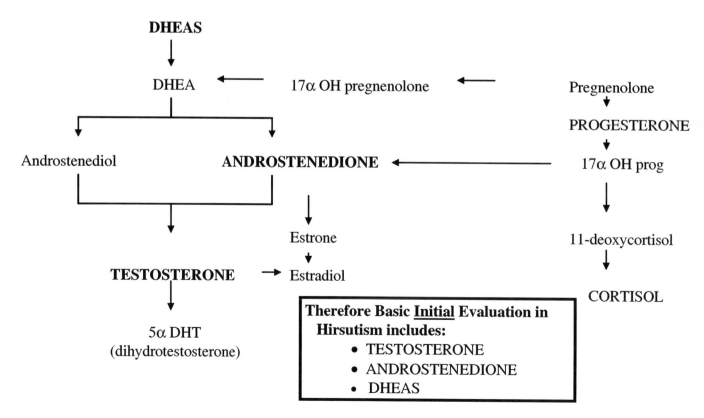

DHEAS

DHEA ← 17α OH pregnenolone ← Pregnenolone

PROGESTERONE

Androstenediol   **ANDROSTENEDIONE** ← 17α OH prog

Estrone   11-deoxycortisol

TESTOSTERONE → Estradiol   CORTISOL

5α DHT
(dihydrotestosterone)

Therefore Basic <u>Initial</u> Evaluation in Hirsutism includes:
- TESTOSTERONE
- ANDROSTENEDIONE
- DHEAS

Subsequent Testing Can Include...
1. LH, FSH, SHBG (Sex hormone-binding globulin)
2. Free Testosterone
3. DHT
4. Estradiol
5. Prolactin
6. ACTH
7. Cortisol
8. Dexamethosone Suppression Testing
9. Trasvaginal U/S

CAH (CONGENITAL ADRENAL HYPERPLASIA)

- *Must know these clinical associations...*

> ✪ **HTN** ←——→ **17 α hydroxylase** deficiency [think of a "hyper" teenager (17)]
> ✪ **Virilization** ←——→ **21-hydroxylase** deficiency; most common (95%) form of CAH.

- ***SEE FIG. 3 APPENDIX***

ORAL CONTRACEPTIVES

- Can be either a combination of estrogen + progestin, *or* progestin only.

- They work by inhibiting GnRH secretion and the mid-cycle LH surge so that ovulation does not occur.

- *Potential complications...*
    1. Migraine

    2. HTN

    3. Hepatic adenoma

    4. ↑ risk of thromboembolism, CAD, CVA

- *Precautions...*(use carefully in these individuals)
    1. Obese

    2. Smokers

    3. Varicose veins

    4. h/o hypercoaguability

ALGORTHMIC APPROACH TO WORKUP ...

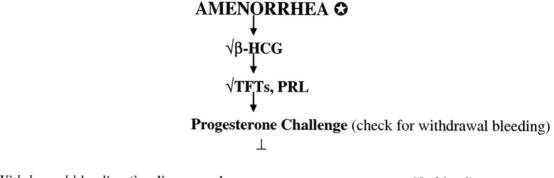

AMENORRHEA ✪

√β-HCG

√TFTs, PRL

Progesterone Challenge (check for withdrawal bleeding)
⊥

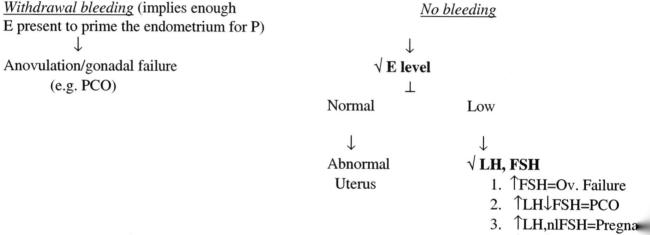

Withdrawal bleeding (implies enough   *No bleeding*
E present to prime the endometrium for P)
↓   ↓
Anovulation/gonadal failure   **√ E level**
(e.g. PCO)   ⊥

Normal   Low

↓   ↓
Abnormal   **√ LH, FSH**
Uterus   1. ↑FSH=Ov. Failure
                2. ↑LH↓FSH=PCO
                3. ↑LH,nlFSH=Pregna
                4. ↓LH↓FSH=Hypopi

Hypopituitarism

- Remember, in treating patients with both ACTH and TSH deficiencies, ***give the glucocorticoid fir*** since supplementing the thyroxine first may exacerbate the need for cortisol and precipate an acute adrenocortical crisis.

Pituitary Tumors

- **There are 4 ways to classify pituitary tumors**
    - i)   "Microadenomas" are < 10mm vs. "macroadenomas" >10mm
    - ii) Sellar vs. extrasellar
    - iii) Functioning vs. non-functioning
    - iv) Isolated vs. part of a MEN I syndrome (multiple endocrine neoplasia type I; MEN I als includes: pancreatic ca and hyperparathyroidism 2° to hyperplastic parathyroid tumor.

- Prolactin-producing tumors are the most common among the functioning tumors.

- Treatment…
    1. Transphenoidal surgery is the operation of choice for most tumors
    2. XRT may also be used as adjuvant/neoadjuvant therapy
    3. Drug therapy with Bromocriptine (a Dopamine agonist) is useful for prolactinomas and GH-producing tumors
    4. Octreotide® (a somatostatin analogue) has also been used.

Prolactinomas
- *Manifest as…*
    1. Amenorrhea/galactorrhea in women
    2. *Decreased libido and potency in men*
        - *These symptoms are often dismissed/passed off as psychiatric factors, thus delaying the diagnosis in men.*
    3. Delayed sexual maturation in adolescents

- *Diagnosis*
    1. In women, always R/O pregnancy first
    2. Check serum PRL (prolactin) level. If the level is >10x normal (>250ng/ml), it establishes the dx of prolactinoma. If <250, R/O functional causes…
        - (a) Drugs
        - (b) 1° hypothyroidism
        - (c) CRF

- *Treatment*
    1. Indicated for management of…
        - (a) Infertility
        - (b) Hypogonadism
        - (c) Significant galactorrhea
        - (d) Hirsutism
    2. *Microprolactinomas*(<10mm, as measured by CT or MRI)→ bromocryptine (dopamine agonist that ↓ tumor size) **or** Transphenoidal surgery.
    3. *Macroprolactinomas*(>10mm)→Surgery is usually not sufficient, so is often combined with either bromocryptine or XRT.

Acromegaly ✪

Clinical Presentation (2° to GH/IGF-1 excess):
1. Acromegalic features
2. *Carbohydrate intolerance* in 20%
3. ↑ Sweating and oily Skin; skin tags
4. ↓ Heat tolerance
5. Acroparesthesias
6. *Carpal tunnel* dz and other Nerve entrapment syndromes
7. Prolactinemia (in up to half the cases), causing amenorrhea/↓libido/galactorrhea
8. *Proximal myopathy*

9. Acanthosis Nigricans (other causes of A.N. are obesity; DM; gastric ca)
10. Sleep apnea
11. Cardiomyopathy or HTN

> ✪ *Remember* → *"PM SNAC"* (**P**rolactinemia/**P**roximal **M**yalgia; **S**weating/oily **S**kin/**S**kin tags; **S**leep apnea; **N**europathies (entrapment);**A**cromegalic features/**A**croparesthesias; **A**canthosis Nigricans; **C**arbohydrate intolerance/**C**ardiomyopathy)

DIAGNOSIS is either by:
1. ↑ *Serum IGF-1 (somatomedin); or*
2. OGTT *(oral glucose tolerance test), checking for non-suppressible GH*, i.e. GH that remains ↑ after administering ↑glucose load(this is the standard reference test). If GH does not suppress to < 10ug/L, the test is positive for GH excess.

MORTALITY is ↑ 2° to:
1. HTN
2. DM
3. Cardiovascular effects

DIABETES INSIPIDUS ✪

1. Causes polyuria and polydipsia (often with preference for ice-cold water); nocturia common.
2. May result from…
   a. <u>Production</u> of AVP→central DI→e.g. breast/lung ca mets, with ***abrupt*** onset of symptoms.
   b. <u>Sensitivity</u> of the kidneys to AVP→nephrogenic DI→e.g. ***Lithium*** toxicity
   c. Functional suppression of AVP →primary <u>polydipsia (compulsive water drinking)</u>→e.g. a ***psych***iatric patient.
3. **Water Deprivation Test**
   a. *Deprive the patient of water and measure the subsequent urine and plasma osmolality.* <u>Normally</u>, this would cause an individual to secrete ADH to conserve their water, causing <u>elevations in subsequent measurements of serum and urine concentration.</u> But in DI, their is either not enough ADH released from the brain or a lack of responsiveness to ADH at the level of the kidneys, so concentrations will not ↑ as expected to.
   b. Therefore, if the urine osm does not ↑ by >10%, the test is positive (for DI).
4. ***Then, may test with exogenous AVP to further clarify the source of the DI only if:***
   a. Sequential urine osm vary by < 30 mosm /kg; or
   b. There is a 3-5% weight loss.

Water deprivation	Response to AVP	DIAGNOSIS
Normal	Absent	1° Polydipsia
+	**Present**	Central DI
+	**Absent**	Nephrogenic DI

5. ***Treatment depends on the cause...***
   a. Central DI→intranasal dDAVP (desmopressin)
   b. Partial central DI→Chlorpropamide (AVP agonist)
   c. Nephrogenic DI→Thiazides, but patient ***must be on a Na+ restricted diet*** to work

SIADH (Syndrome of Inappropriate ADH Secretion)

1. Relatively hypoosmolar serum; relatively hyperosmolar urine
2. ↑ **Urine Na (>30)**
3. ↓ serum Na+ ; a ↓ serum Uric acid is also a frequent concomitant.
4. To make this diagnosis, you *must first rule out* the following conditions...
   a. ↑ or ↓ volume (SIADH is a euvolemic state)
   b. Effect of diuretics
   c. Thyroid deficiency (√TSH)
   d. Adrenal deficiency (√ACTH)
5. Treatment
   a. Best treatment for the ↓ serum Na+ is **water restriction**.
   b. If the patient has **symptomatic** ↓Na+ with neurologic sequelae, then **hypertonic saline** is the tx.
   c. It is said that overly rapid correction of the serum Na+ with hypertonic saline can lead to CPM (Central Pontine Myelinolysis).

THYROID DISORDERS

⊗ **THE RELATIONSHIP BETWEEN GOITERS AND THYROIDITIS :**
(either can also be thyrotoxic or underactive) :

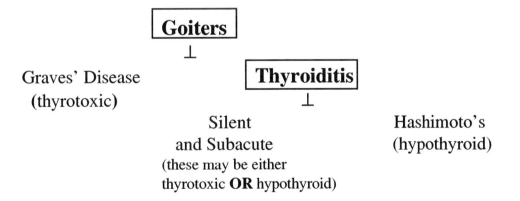

| **Goiters** |
| ⊥ |

Graves' Disease
(thyrotoxic)   **Thyroiditis**
                           ⊥

Silent   Hashimoto's
and Subacute   (hypothyroid)
(these may be either
thyrotoxic **OR** hypothyroid)

- ***THYROID SCANNING*** (24 hour **Iodine** [131] **uptake**)
  - Useful in the DDx of **THYROTOXICOSIS WITH DIFFUSE GOITER...**

    ⊗ ↑UPTAKE→**Graves' Disease**
    ⊗ ↓UPTAKE→**Subacute and silent thyroiditis**

DIFFERENTIATING THYROIDITIS:

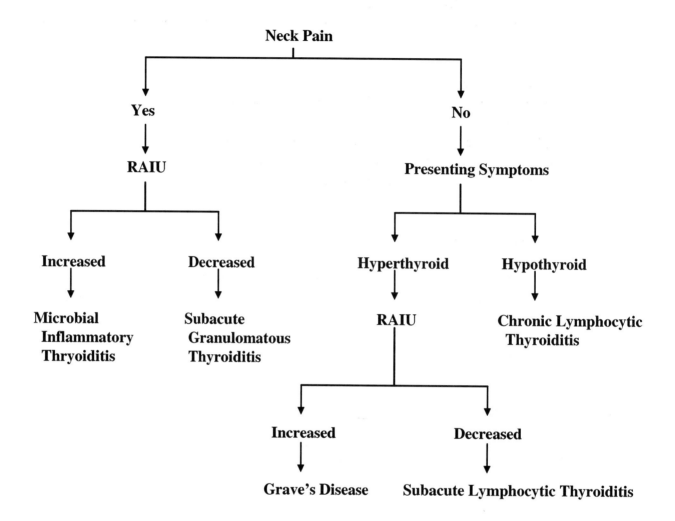

THYROIDITIS TERMS/SYNONYMS:

Chronic Lymphocytic Thyroiditis	aka **Hashimoto's** thyroiditis
Subacute Thyroiditis	Re: tender, *painful*; usually *viral* etiology
Silent Thyroiditis	Re: *painless*; lymphocytic; *postpartum*
Granulomatous	aka Subacute granulomatous thyroiditis; de Quervain's
Microbial inflammatory	Suppurative thyroiditis; acute thyroiditis
Invasive fibrous	Riedel's struma; Riedel's thyroiditis.

Subacute & Silent Thyroiditis (can be ↑ or ↓ thyroid)

◆ Inflamed/damaged thyroid tissue causes release of stored hormones→a few weeks of mild **thyrotoxicosis that may be followed by** a short period of **hypothyroidism** while the thyroid recovers.

◆ **2 types (both self-limiting):**

1. **SUBACUTE**
   a) Uncommon
   b) Painful, *tender* goiter
   c) Causative agent felt to be <u>viral</u>
   d) ↑*thyroglobulin;* ↑*temp;* ↑*ESR;* ↓ I uptake
   e) Self-limiting
   f) For moderate disease→may treat with NSAIDs
   g) For more severe disease→may treat with prednisone

2. **Painless lymphocytic; so-called "SILENT"**
   a) Common
   b) Acute (often postpartum), transient thyrotoxicosis usual
   c) Self-limiting disease, but a tendency to recur ; beta-blockers prn
   d) Normal ESR

✪ *REMEMBER,* **the #1 cause of <u>Hyper</u>thyroidism is** *Graves'* **Disease, and the #1 cause of hypothyroidism is** *Hashimoto's* **thyroiditis. <u>Therefore</u>,** the #1 cause of both is an <u>*autoimmune*</u> disorder.

Hypothyroidism (Hashimoto's Thyroiditis)
1. Also the most common form of thyroiditis
2. **Anti-microsomal Ab** is usually present; **Antithyroglobulin Ab** present over ½ the time.
3. Clinical
   a) Bradycardia
   b) Constipation
   c) Carpal tunnel syndrome
   d) Pericardial/pleural effusions
   e) Associated autoimmune disorders (e.g. DM)
   f) Hyperlipidemia
   g) HTN; cardiomyopathy

4. May present with *<u>lymphocytic thyroiditis</u>* (*postpartum* transient hyperthyroidism followed by transient hypothyroidism as is seen within 6 months of delivery.) Antimicrosomal Ab is usually +.
5. May be goitrous or atrophic.

Hyperthyroidism

1. *Main causes include…*
   a) Nodular goiter—
   b) Single (Toxic Nodular Goiter, or TNG) *or*
   c) Multiple (Toxic Multinodular Goiter, or TMG—below)
   d) Thyroiditis—silent or subacute
   e) Graves' disease
   f) Tumors

2. ## Graves' Disease
   a) **2 types of ocular findings** ✪
      (1) Infiltrative findings (only Graves'):
         (a) Proptosis
         (b) Optic neuritis
         (c) Extraocular muscle dysfunction
      (2) Noninfiltrative Findings (any thyrotoxicosis)
         (a) Lid lag
         (b) Lid retraction
   b) Diffuse goiter
   c) Thyrotoxicosis 2° to *thyroid-stimulating antibodies*
   d) 20% of patients, especially elderly, may not evince goiter

3. ## Diffuse Goiter
   a) *Graves's Disease*
      (1) ↓sTSH
      (2) ↑Iodine uptake
   b) *Silent Thyroiditis*
      (1) ↓TSH
      (2) ↓ Iodine uptake

4. ## Toxic Multinodular Goiter (TMG)
   a) A disease of the elderly
   b) An *"apathetic" hyperthyroid* ✪ (note the oxymoron) (may mimic depression); picture dominates with…
      (1) Weakness
      (2) Loss of appetite
      (3) Loss of energy
      (4) Cardiovascular effects (arrythmias;CHF)

5. ## Toxic Nodular Goiter (TNG)
   a) Solitary nodule > 3cm
   b) Isolated intense ↑ uptake on thyroid scan

6. **Thyroiditis**—previously discussed—remember: can be ↓ or↑ thyroid

7. **Factitious Thyrotoxicosis**
   i)   Ingested T3 or T4
   ii)   Suspect it in thyrotoxic individuals with all of the following…
       a)   High T4 or T3
       b)   **No** goiter
       c)   ↓ TSH
       d)   ↓ serum thyroglobulin
       e)   ↓ I-131 UPTAKE

8. **Treatment**…
   i)   <u>**BY DISEASE:**</u>

       a)   *Graves*→<u>RAI</u> (Radioactive Iodine)---If patient is pregnant, surgery (subtotal thyroidectomy) or antithyroid meds—see below—are appropriate treatment alternatives to RAI.

       b)   *TNG*→<u>RAI</u> or surgery

       c)   *TMG*→<u>RAI</u> or surgery

          •   Remember, ***pregnancy*** is the only absolute contraindication to RAI; the only major drawback of RAI is the development of hypothyroidism

       d)   *Silent Thyroiditis*→symptomatic/supportive since self-remitting

       e)   *Subacute Thyroiditis*→as per silent thyroiditis + steroids/NSAIDs

       f)   Tumor→surgery

   ii)   **ANTITHYROID MEDICATION**

       a)   **Methimazole**--↓ T4 production

       b)   **Propylthiouracil (PTU)**--↓ T4 production <u>& blocks T4→T3</u> conversion
       c)   Side effects of these agents…
          (1)   Agranulocytosis
          (2)   Aplastic Anemia
          (3)   Hepatitis
          (4)   Vasculitis

       d) Beta-Blockers should be considered as adjunctive treatment only.

ALGORITHMIC WORKUP OF A THYROID NODULE...

FINE NEEDLE ASPIRATION:

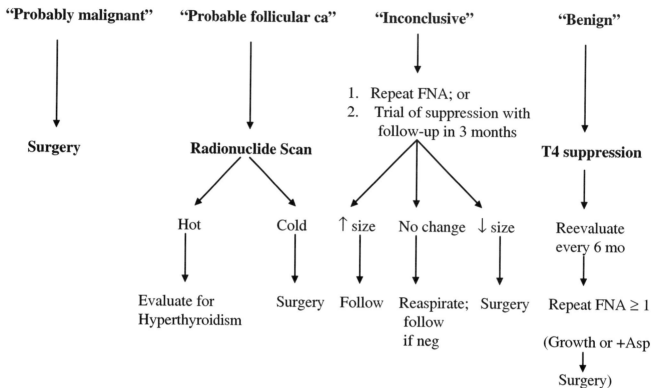

Thryoid nodules

90% rule of thumb:
- 90% are benign
- 90% (!) are "cold" (Note: only 20% of these are actually malignant; 1% for hot nodules)
- 90% are solid

THYROID CA ✪

1. Nevertheless, remember, the classic link "**C** old" nodule↔**C** ancer.
2. "Hot" nodules→nearly always benign
3. **Papillary ca** is the most common and has the *best prognosis*. It *spreads via lymph*
4. *nodes*, and can present with thryoid mass and + cervical LNs.
5. **Follicular ca**—spreads *hematogenously*
6. **Anaplastic ca**
   a. Seen mostly in the elderly
   b. *Very aggressive*
   c. *Worst prognosis*
7. **Medullary ca**
   a. *Calcitonin* is the tumor marker
   b. Amyloid deposits common
   c. May be isolated or part of MEN IIA or IIB, so *should therefore R/O pheo and hyperparathyroidism (IIA)*

Euthyroid Sick Syndrome ✪
1. Aka "Adaptive hypothyroidism"
2. Seen in hospitalized patients (thus "euthyroid sick")
3. ↓T3 ↓T4 ↓sTSH (therefore **can look like Central Hypothyroidism**, except may also see ↑*cortisol* levels from); *free T4 is normal*; ↑ reverse T3.
4. Because of the ↓sTSH, sTSH should not be used alone to screen for thyroid dz in hospitalized patients.
5. The condition is primarily a laboratory phenomenon, is only a reflection of the patient's generally ill condition, and warrants no additional treatment.

Thyroid Disease and Pregnancy
Normal Pregnant State
1. ↑T3 and ↑T4 2° to estrogen-induced ↑ in TBG
2. FTI unchanged
3. *Neither RAI nor Beta-blockers should be given.* B-blockers can result in…
   a. Fetal growth retardation
   b. Neonatal respiratory depression

Graves' Disease
1. Antithyroid drug therapy is the rule even these drugs cross the placenta
2. *Surgery is considered a viable option in the **second** trimester.* ✪

Thyrotoxic Crisis:
1. Untreated or inadequately treated **HYPER**thyroid patients undergoing surgical treatment or who have another acute illness
2. Clinical:
   a. ↑ Temp; ↑ Pulse; ↓ BP
   b. Vomiting/diarrhea
   c. Irritability; delirium
   d. coma and even death if untreated
3. PTU, Na Iodide, and Propranolol are used to control the crisis
   • Remember, PTU blocks the <u>synthesis</u> of thyroxine, and Na Iodide blocks the <u>release</u> of thyroxine from the thyroid

Myxedema Crisis: (Don't confuse: the physical sign of myxedema is seen in thyrotoxicosis!)
1. Occurs in severe **HYPO**thyroidism
2. While it may occur spontaneously, it can be brought on by illness, cold, physiologic stressors.
3. 20-50% mortality
4. Clinical:
   a. ↓: Temp/BP/Resp/Na/Glucose
   b. Gradual onset with lethargy→stupor→*coma*
5. Treatment
   ✪ *Aggressive IV thyroxine repletion;*
   ✪ *High dose steroids*

Parathyroid Disease
Remember…
1. *Magnesium* is necessary for PTH secretion.
2. Serum Ca is the key controlling factor for PTH secretion
3. The best PTH to order is an ***Intact PTH***
4. Vit D comes from diet and from photogenesis of vit D precursors in the skin.

1° HYPERparathyroidism
[**See Figure 1 (Appendix):** <u>**ALGORITHMIC APPROACH TO ↑SERUM CA:**</u>]

1. Usually from an ***adenoma*** (not hyperplasia); adenoma is solitary 80% of the time
2. Hyperplasia only 15% of the time (e.g. in MEN I, IIA)
3. Carcinoma only 2% of the time
4. May be part of ***MEN I or IIA; these types are hyperplastic*** lesions.
5. Usually asymptomatic; however, if you see a hypercalcemic patient with ***HTN and renal stones*** or chondrocalcinosis/pseudogout→ think hyperparathyroidism→ √ an *intact PTH*
6. Additional skeletal lesions that can be found include…
    a. Periosteal bone resorption e.g. at the distal phalanges
    b. Ostitis fibrosis cystica
    c. Salt and pepper lesions seen on skull plain film
7. The key differential diagnosis is FHH (Familial Hypocalciuric Hypercalcemia), another cause of ↑ serum Ca. The way to DDx these is by *√ **Urine Ca. It's low in FHH***; normal to ↑ in 1° hyperpara.
8. ↑ PTH. If the PTH is ↓, must consider parathyroid-independent hyperCa (tumors; sarcoid; vit D intox; etc).
9. Treatment is surgery.

Familial Hypocalciuric Hypercalcemia (FHH)
1. Autosomal dominant hyperCa in a relatively young patient
2. PTH is ↔ to slightly ↑, and therefore, cannot be used to DDx with 1° hyperpara, so check the Urine Ca.
3. Important in the differential of hyperpara since diagnosis precludes parathyroidectomy!
4. A benign condition; no treatment necessary.

♦ **Thiazides → Cause mild ↑serum Ca; and ↓ Urine Ca (unlike other diuretics).**
♦ **Lithium → Causes ↑ serum Ca in 10% since it ↑'s the setpoint of PTH secretion.**

✪ *Remember* → **FHH, thiazides, and Lithium** are common causes of "normal" or "minimally elevated" PTH.

Hypercalcemia of Malignancy

1. *Statistically is the #1 cause of ↑Ca in hospitalized patients.*

2. *Many mechanisms depending on the tumor…*

   ✪ *Multiple Myeloma→↑OAF (Osteoclast Activating Factor)→bone resorption*
   ✪ *Lymphoma and Sarcoidosis→ ectopic production of 1,25 Vit D*
   ✪ *PTH-rP (PTH-related Protein)*—humoral hyperCa of malignancy
      (i) Squamous cell ca of lung, head, and neck; and
      (ii) Ca of breast/kidney/GU tract.

Treatment of Hypercalcemic Disorders:

1. Volume repletion first →THEN forced saline diuresis

2. Inhibitors of osteoclastic activity (i.e. of bone resorption; *Remember*: Osteo**B**lasts **B**uild; Osteo**C**lasts **C**hew up bone):

   a) Calcitonin—can see Tachyphylaxis
   b) Bisphosphonates (e.g. Etidronate; Palmidronate)
   c) Gallium Nitrate

♦ **Remember→ ↑ Ca^{2+} in Addison's, vit D intoxication, and sarcoidosis are steroid-responsive.**

HYPOparathyroidism

1. ↓ Serum Ca
2. Clinical:
      a) Cardiovascular--↑ QTc; CHF
      b) GI—Abdominal pain; N/V
      c) Neuromuscular—paresthesias; muscle spasms; Chvostek's and Trousseau's signs.
      d) Neurologic—basal ganglia calcification; benign intracranial HTN

3. *Remember to first RULE OUT…*
      a) *↓Mg: a common cause of hypopara, since Mg needed for PTH secretion and action*
      b) Low serum Albumin. If albumin, calculate the corrected Ca or order an ionized Ca.
         Re: **Corrected Ca**= measured Ca + [(4-measured albumin)x0.8]
      c) Renal insufficiency

4. ***Remember, just as*** HYPERpara can be 1°, 2°, and 3°, so HYPO para can be…
   a) **Hypopara-- ↓ PTH**
   b) **"Pseudo" hypopara—↑PTH** (r/o ↓ vit D and renal failure); genetic;
      2° to **end-organ resistance to PTH; urinary cAMP is ↓**

   Clinical—may see…
   - (i)   Short stature/short neck/short metacarpals
   - (ii)   Rounded face/obesity/mild mental retardation
   - (iii) SQ Calcification

   c) **"Pseudopseudo"** hypopara—same as (b) **but without the biochemical markers.**

5. **Treatment**
   Correct any readily identifiable cause:
   - If life-threatening, give Ca supplementation intravenously
   - Oral phospate binders may be useful as well as thiazides to ↓ urinary Ca excretion.

✪ MEN I Syndrome (Multiple Endocrine Neoplasia)—aka Wermer Syndrome

1. Pituitary tumors
2. <u>Parathyroid tumor</u>
3. Pancreatic ca

✪ MEN IIA Syndrome—aka Sipple Syndrome

1. Pheo—remember, you have "**II**" adrenals (and in fact, the pheo in Sipple's in usually bilateral)
2. <u>Parathyroid tumor</u>
3. Medullary thyroid ca

DIABETES

CRITERIA FOR DIAGNOSING DIABETES				
<u>Test</u>	**Results**			
	Normal	**IFG**[1]	**IGT**[2]	**Diabetes**
Fasting glucose	<110	110-125		126
Glucose intolerance (2h after 75g glucose load)	<140		140-199	200
Random glucose				200 with symptoms

[1] IFG, impaired fasting glucose
[2] IGT, impaired glucose intolerance

✪ *The new cutoff for diagnosis is FBS $\geq$ 126.*

● *Ideally, FBS should be <115*

● *A1C% (Normal is < 6%); Goal is < 7%; >8% is certainly an indication for action.*

● Note, 70-85% of **NIDDM** patients are usually **obese**

SOMOGYI EFFECT vs. DAWN PHENOMENON !

✪ *Somogyi effect= Rebound hyperglycemia* 2° to counter-regulatory hormones
(such as GH) that follows a hypoglycemic episode.
Treatment is to *decrease* the patient's insulin.

✪ *Dawn phenomenon*=↑ early AM glusoses 2° to insulin resistance.
Treatment is to *increase* the patient's insulin.

NOTE*: Both of these early am phenomona are hyperglycemic in
nature, yet the treatments are exact opposites. Usually, the dawn
phenomenon can be differentiated from posthypoglycemic
hyperglycemia (Somogyi) by measuring the blood glucose at 3 A.M*

| TREATMENT GOALS FOR DIABETICS ||
PARAMETER	GOAL
Blood Glucose	
Fasting blood sugar	<120 mg/dl
1h postprandial	<180
Hgb A1C	<7.0%
Lipids	
Total Cholesterol	<200
LDL	<100
HDL	>42 males; >35 females
TG	<150
Blood Pressure	<130/85
Healthy **Weight** (based on BMI, body mass index)	Normal BMI < 25 Overweight: BMI 25-29.9 Obesity: BMI ≥30

CLASSES OF AGENTS FOR USE IN TYPE 2 DM HYPERGLYCEMIA

AGENT	PRIMARY ACTION
Thiazolidinediones (rosiglitazone, pioglitazone)	Bind to peroxisome-proliferator-activated receptor-gamma (PPAR-gamma) in muscle, fat, and liver to ↓ insulin resistance
Insulin secretagogues [e.g. sulfonylureas (gliburide, glipizide), repaglinide]	Stimulate pancreatic beta cells to ↑ insulin output.
Biguanides (e.g. metformin)	Liver: ↓ glucose production Muscle: ↑ glucose uptake
Alpha-glucosidase inhibitors (e.g. acarbose, miglitol)	Inhibit intestinal enzymes that break down carbohydrates, thus delaying carbohydrate absorption
Insulins	Target insulin-sensitive tissue to ↑glucose uptake

DIABETIC EYE DISEASE

✪ A. *BACKROUND RETINOPATHY*

1. "Dot and blot" intraretinal **hemorrhages**
2. **Exudates** are either…
   - (a) "Cotton wool" spots (microinfarcts of superficial retina); or
   - (b) "Hard" exudates, from protein/lipids leaking from capillaries of deep
     retinal layers
3. **Microaneurysms**

✪ B. *PROLIFERATIVE RETINOPATHY*

- In 10-15%, **proliferative** retinopathy develops 2° to underlying retinal ischemia that leads to new vessel formation.

- *Complications of proliferative retinopathy to remember include:*

   - (a) *Vitreous hemorrhages*
   - (b) *Retinal detachment*
   - (c) *Neovascularization*

- Proliferative retinopathy may therefore present as *sudden monocular visual loss*
- Proliferative retinopathy is the chief cause of blindness ages 20-64

C. *MACULOPATHY* (chief cause of blindness in DM): edema/exudates/ischemia

D. And remember, there's an ↑frequency of cataracts and glaucoma in diabetics

DIABETIC RENAL DISEASE
1. *Microalbumin*, defined as 30-250mg/24h, precedes overt proteinuria and identifies patients at risk for nephropathy; therefore it is an important screening test in diabetics.
2. If microalbumin is detected, an ACE inhibitor can be started to slow down/halt the progression of proteinuria and decrease one's risk of developing nephropathy
3. *ACE inhibitors* are also 1st line therapy in HTN + DM with normal renal function.
4. Contrast dyes may precipitate renal failure, depending on other risk factors, including old age, dehydration, liver disease, and preexisting renal dz.
5. *Kimmelstiel-Wilson* kidneys seen on pathology and represent progression of renal disease.
✪ **Hypo**reninemic **hypo**aldosteronism is the type 4 RTA of DM.

DIABETIC NEUROPATHY
1. **Peripheral polyneuropathy** is most commonly seen
   a) Usually bilateral, symmetric—so-called "stocking-glove" distribution
   b) Paresthesias, numbness, hyperesthesia, or deep pain worse at night

2. **Mononeuropathy**
   a) Etiology most likely vascular
   b) Commonly spontaneously remit
   c) Clinically may see…
      (1) Footdrop (*isolated peroneal neuropathy*)
      (2) Sudden wristdrop
      (3) Painful diplopia 2° to dysfunction of cranial nerves 3/4/6
3. **Autonomic** Neuropathy
   a) Constipation most common, but can also see diarrhea
   b) Diabetic *gastroparesis*—important 2° to potential unpredictable swings in plasma glucose.

4. Diabetic neuropathies may also be classified as follows:
   a) **Diffuse neuropathies** (generally more common, progressive, and more insidious in onset)
      (1) Distal symmetrical sensorimotor polyneuropathy
      (2) Autonomic neuropathy
   b) **Focal neuropathies** (generally more rare, more sudden in onset, and more transient)
      (1) Radiculopathy
      (2) Mononeuropathy/ mononeuropathy multiplex
         (a) Entrapment neuropathy
         (b) Other mononeuropathies
      (3) Plexopathy
      (4) Cranial nerve palsies

DIABETIC AMYOTROPHY
1. Progressive *weakness, pain, atrophy* of the pelvic girdle and anterior thigh muscles.
2. Spontaneously abates after 6-12 months

Metformin (Glucophage®)

1. Predominant antihyperglycemic effect is in ↓*ing hepatic glucose production*, although it als[?] works to ↑*glucose uptake* at the muscle
2. Important Contraindications for the exam…
   - a) ↑Creatinine:
     - (1) **Males: creat ≥ 1.5**
     - (2) **Females: creat ≥ 1.4**
   - b) Abnormal liver function or alcohol abuse
   - c) Chronic acidosis or hypoxia

Sulfonylureas

- These <u>primarily</u> act to ↑ *the ability of the pancreas to secrete insulin*, but also work to greater *sensitize the peripheral tissues to insulin.*
- Remember, *Chlorpropamide*, one of the older agents still occasionally seen may cause *SIADH*.

- **Contraindications**…
  1. Pregnant/lactating diabetics
  2. Sulfa allergy
  3. Hepatic/renal baseline abnormality

- Because of the relatively long half lives of some of these agents, there is a greater risk of developing hypoglycemia, esp in elderly who are either malnourished or have baseline liver/kidney dysfunction.

DKA (Diabetic Ketoacidosis)

1. *Seen in Type I diabetes only (Type II diabetes can have Hyperosmolar Nonketotic Coma, HONC)*
   - *In general, blood glucose and volume deficits are much higher in HONC tha[n] in DKA. Patients with DKA are usually 4-6L behind (versus 8-10L in HONC[)]*
2. *Characterized by…*
   - a) Insulin deficiency
   - b) ↑Glucose
   - c) Dehydration 2° osmotic diuresis
   - d) Ketonemia
   - e) Metabolic acidosis

3. **Common** *Symptoms*
   - a) Abdominal pain
   - b) Anorexia
   - c) Change in vision
   - d) Fatigue
   - e) Nausea and vomiting
   - f) Thirst and polyuria
   - g) Weakness

4. **Common *Signs***
    a)   Dehydration
    b)   Hyperventilation
    c)   Hypotension
    d)   Impaired consciousness and/or coma
    e)   Tachycardia
    f)   Warm, dry skin
    g)   Weight loss

5. ***Typical Laboratories***
    a)   Arterial pH <7.2 (also the level below which supplemental bicarbonate is indicated)
    b)   Plasma bicarbonate ≤15meq/L
    c)   Blood glucose ≥250mg/dl
    d)   Ketones + in the blood and urine

6. ***Precipitating factors*** for DKA include most any major physiologic stressor, e.g....
    a)   CVA
    b)   Emotional stress
    c)   Infection
    d)   MI (thereofore an EKG is indicated in all adult patients)
    e)   Noncompliance with insulin regimen

✪   As you correct the metabolic acidosis and hyperglycemia, ***serum K+*** ↓, so remember to add KCl to your IVF when K+ drops. Remember the ***inverse correlation*** between serum K+ and pH. That's why ***Bicarbonate*** is given with ↑ serum K+. Speaking of Bicarb, it should only be added if pH <7.2

✪   Remember, DKA patients are ***deficient in total body K+*** regardless of their plasma K+ concentration.

✪   ***Remember to switch*** from IV insulin to SQ when serum glucose ↓s to 200-250

✪   The best way to monitor a patient with DKA for improvement is ***serial Anion Gaps***, and *not* urine ketones.

HONC (Hyperosmolar Nonketotic Coma)

1. Very high glucoses with significant osmotic (thus HONC) diuresis. Consequently, these patients need even more ***aggressive IVFluid resuscitation***. Start with Normal Saline to correct the volume deficit→then switch to ½ NS to correct the hyperosmolarity

2. ***No ketoacidosis*** (thus HONC) since enough insulin is available to inhibit ketone production.

3. Seen only in ***Type II DM***

COMPLICATIONS OF INSULIN RESISTANCE
1. Hyperinsulinemia associated with:
    a. Atherogenesis
    b. HTN
    c. Dyslipidemia
2. Hyperglycemia and relative insulin deficiency…

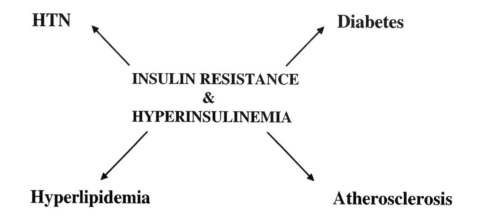

PREGNANCY AND DIABETES

1. ***Tight control*** of sugars in preexisting diabetic during pregnancy is important

    a)   If poor control in ***first trimester***→ ↑ risk of congenital malformations
    b)   If poor control in ***2nd/3rd trimesters***→ ↑ risk of …
        (1)   Macrosomia
        (2)   Neonatal ↓glu, ↓Ca, ↑RBCs, ↑bili,
        (3)   Resp distress

2. As sulfonylureas are contraindicated, ***insulin*** therapy is the treatment.

3. Advanced maternal age is a risk factor for gestational DM.

4. Gestational DM is itself a risk factor for ***future development of Type II DM*** (50-60% risk over the ensuing 15 years)

Insulinomas
1. Not unlike pheo (!), there is a rule of 10's…
    a)   10% are multiple
    b)   10% are malignant
    c)   10% are MEN I - related
2. Rare islet-cell tumor
3. Important in the DDx of hypoglycemia

[See Figure 2:   **LABORATORY EVALUATION OF HYPOGLYCEMIA**]

ADRENOCORTICAL FAILURE

[See Figure 3 for <u>Synthesis Pathways of Cortisol,Testosterone, & Aldosterone</u>]

1. *↓ Aldosterone and ↓ cortisol* which lead to the following clinical picture:

   a) Weakness; fatigue
   b) ↓Appetite
   c) ↓BP
   d) ↓ Glucose
   e) ↓Na+
   f) ↑Pigment (e.g. at the palmar creases)
   g) ↑K+

2. Causes of ↓ aldo for the boards…

   1° Failure (Addison's Disease)—*these patients have <u>hyperreninemic hypoaldosteronism.</u>*

   a) *Autoimmune is the #1 cause*
   b) TB; fungal disorders;
   c) Malignancy

   ✪ *Waterhouse-Friederickson Syndrome (bilateral adrenal hemorrhage) 2° to sepsis (e.g. meningococcal)*, trauma, anticoagulants--#2 cause in the US.

   2° Failure (most patients)

   a) Following removal of adrenal tumor—may take up to 1 year for the HPA axis to recover.
   b) NSAIDs
   c) ACE inhibitors

   ✪ *Prolonged steroid use* (suppresses ACTH)--#1 cause of 2° failure

3. Frequent association of antithyroid antibodies in autoimmune Addison's.

✪ Diagnosis: ***Cosyntropin test***. This test checks the cortisol response after infusing Cosyntropin (an ACTH analogue). A subnormal cortisol response indicates adrenocortical failure (although it doesn't differentiate 1° vs. 2° causes—*ACTH levels* do that). A normal response excludes it.

---

4. *The treatment differs for 1° vs 2° Adrenocortical failure*.

   • 1°→Glucocorticoid (hydrocortisone) + Mineralcorticoid therapy (fludrocortisone)

   • 2°→Glucocorticoid only

CUSHING'S DISEASE

- ♦ 2° to steroid excess (↑cortisol; opposite of Adrenocortical failure)
- ♦ Actually, the terminology goes…

  a) Cushing's **Disease**=2° disease at the level of the pituitary; caused by ACTH-producing tumor or hyperplasia.
  b) Cushing's **Syndrome**=1° disease at the level of the adrenal.

- ♦ *Etiologies*
  - • *65% Cushing's Disease per se*
  - • *10% Adrenal adenoma*
  - • *10% Adrenal carcinoma*
  - • *15% Ectopic ACTH*
  - • *1% Ectopic CRH*

- ♦ *Clinical* (these are also the potential side effects of long term exogenous steroid use!)

  a) Obesity
  b) HTN; DM
  c) ↑Androgens
  d) Cataracts
  e) Easy bruising
  f) Osteoporosis
  g) Striae (stretch marks)
  h) "Moon face" (rounded face)
  i) "Buffalo hump" (fat pad)

- ✪ **CUSHING'S DDX AND DIAGNOSTICS:**

DIAGNOSIS:	ACTH:	Suppressible with High Dose (8mg) Dexamethasone?
Disease (pituitary level)	↑	Y
Syndrome (adrenal level)	↓	N
Ectopic ACTH (e.g. tumors)	↑	N

- ✪ *A 24 hour urine for free cortisol is the simplest screen for Cushing's syndrome.*

- ✪ **Remember, in DST (Dexamethasone Suppresson Test)…**

  a) **1mg**→is for *screening*; aka "overnight test" *(or can do a 24h urine for free cortisol*
  b) **2mg**→is for *confirmation)*; the 2mg DST is aka "low dose DST"; a 2 day test.
  c) **8mg**→is for *pinpointing* the exact cause; aka "high dose DST"; a 2 day test.

    d) *False Positive test results can be seen with*
- (1) Estrogen or BCPs or pregnancy
- (2) Simple obesity
- (3) Depression
- (4) Alcoholism
- (5) Hospitalized patients

HYPERALDOSTERONISM

- Clinical: <u>**HTN**</u>; ↓K+
- **Primary causes** have ↓*renin*; Similar to hyperpara, most (70%) are adenoma; 30% hyperplasia.; only imaging can differentiate these.
- **Secondary causes** have ↑*renin* and include malignant HTN; renovascular HTN; renal artery stenosis; and renin-secreting tumor

- *Workup* for Hyperaldosteronism:

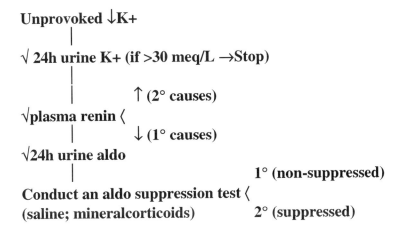

Unprovoked ↓K+

√ **24h urine K+ (if >30 meq/L →Stop)**

         ↑ **(2° causes)**

√**plasma renin** ⟨

         ↓ **(1° causes)**

√**24h urine aldo**

         1° (non-suppressed)

Conduct an aldo suppression test ⟨
(saline; mineralcorticoids)   **2° (suppressed)**

PHEOCHROMOCYTOMA

- <u>**Rule of 10's**</u> (*don't confuse with insulinoma—see above*):
  1. 10% are familial (MEN 2A, 2B)
  2. 10% are extraadrenal
  3. 10% are bilateral
  4. 10% are malignant

- **Clinical** (easy to recall since *all hyperadrenergic symptoms*)
  1. HTN
  2. Orthostatic Hypotension
  3. Headaches 2° to HTN
  4. Tachycardia/palpitations
  5. Sweating
  6. Weight loss

- **Diagnosis via 24 urine for:**

    1. Free catecholamines (Epi; Norepi);

    2. Metanephrines (the metabolites); and

    3. VMA (vanillylmandelic acid)

- **Management**

    1. Surgical excision is curative

    2. MIBG (meta-iodobenzylguanidine) nuclear scans are used to R/O metastatic disease as appropriate.

    3. **Preoperative medical management**:

        ✪ _α blockers, such as phentolamine or phenoxybenzamine, are most important, esp for treating the HTN;_

        ✪ _β blockers (only after adequate α blockade) for any tachyarrhythmias_

"INCIDENTALOMAS" (Incidentally discovered adrenal mass)

- Approx'ly 1 in 10 autopsies

- A little over ½% of all CT scans

- Ca is usually > 4cm; the more common adenomas usually < 6cm

---

✪ _If <4cm and non-hypersecreting, reimage (MRI, CT) in 3 months and periodically thereafter._

✪ _If, on the other hand, the adrenal mass is > 4cm, has grown, or is hypersecreting→it should be excised._

- **Must R/O:**

    1. Pheo → √ <u>24 h urine</u> as above

    2. Cushing's syndrome → √ <u>24 h urine for free cortisol</u>

    3. Primary hyperaldo→ √ <u>Serum K+</u> for starters; then as shown above

    4. Androgen producing tumors→ √ <u>serum DHEAS</u> levels

    5. TB/fungus/carcinoma→ √ <u>CXR</u>

APPENDIX

igure 1. ## ALGORITHMIC APPROACH TO ↑ SERUM CA:

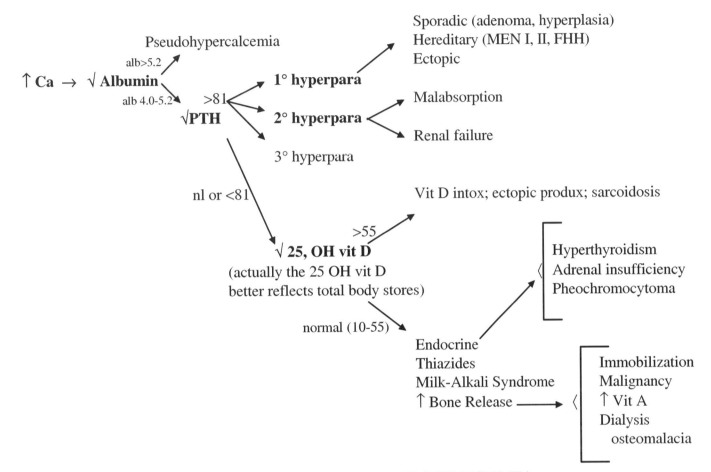

gure 2. ## LABORATORY EVALUATION OF HYPOGLYCEMIA

Diagnosis	Glucose	Insulin	C-peptide	Proinsulin
lfonylurea abuse	↓	↑	↑ *	↔
rreptitious insulin	↓	↑↑	↓**	↓
sulinoma	↓	↑	↑	↑

* <u>High C-peptide</u> implies *endogenous* insulin secretion, which can result from either:
  a) Insulinoma; or
  b) Sulfonylurea abuse—this can be confirmed by simply checking sulfonylurea levels.
  • Consequently, in hyperinsulinemic patients, the exclusion of sulfonylurea abuse
    points to insulinoma. Remember, sulfonylureas ↑ insulin secretion.
** <u>Low C-peptide</u>, on the other hand, implies *exogenous* source, such as surreptious insulin

Figure 3.   SYNTHESIS PATHWAYS OF CORTISOL AND TESTOSTERONE :

a thru c = enzymes, from which you should *know for your exam,*

> **a** =17α-hydroxylase
> **b** =21-hydroxylase
> **c** =11β-hydroxylase

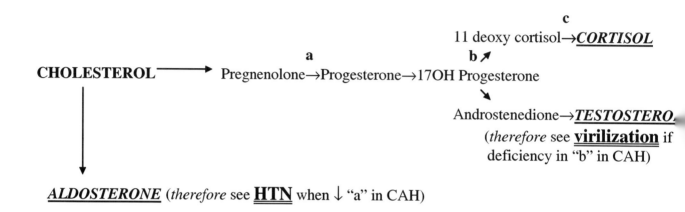

c
11 deoxy cortisol→***CORTISOL***

a   **b** ↗

CHOLESTEROL ———→ Pregnenolone→Progesterone→17OH Progesterone

↘

Androstenedione→***TESTOSTERO***

(*therefore* see **virilization** if
deficiency in "b" in CAH)

ALDOSTERONE (*therefore* see **HTN** when ↓ "a" in CAH)

14. I. NEPHROLOGY
II. CLINICAL TOXICOLOGY

NEPHROLOGY

Commonly Asked Material:

1. RTA's:
   - Type 1 RTA (e.g. Amphotericin B)=distal; $\downarrow$K+
   - Type 2 RTA (e.g. Aminoglycosides)=proximal; $\downarrow$K+
   - Type 4 RTA (e.g. DM; BPH; NSAIDs)=hyporeninemic hypoaldosteronism (hypo hypo); $\uparrow$K+

2. Know that *microalbuminuria* in a diabetic (with or without e.g. borderline HTN) is an indication for ACE Inhibitors (e.g. lisinopril and enalapril)

3. Usually by the time a diabetic has developed microalbuminuria, s/he has developed signs of retinopathy.

4. In slowing the rate of progression of diabetic nephropathy, achieve good BP control (an ACE I would also accomplish this) and shoot for good glucose control.

5. Nephrotic syndrome
   - See >3.5g protein/24h urine; proteinuria$\rightarrow\downarrow$albumin$\rightarrow$edema; $\uparrow$chol
   - proteinuria$\rightarrow$Antithrombin III deficiency(a protein important in anticoag)$\rightarrow$renal vein thrombosis (RVT)$\rightarrow$thrombemboli can be seen$\rightarrow$pulmonary emboli.

6. Know how to calculate the corrected calcium, given the measured calcium and the albumin, and that if the corrected calcium is low, you obviously have to replete.

$$\textit{Corrected Ca}= \text{serum Ca} \; + \; [(4\text{-measured alb})\text{x .8}]$$

7. You must learn the *formula for* glomerular filtration rate:

$$\textbf{GFR}= \frac{(140\text{-age}) \text{ x } \text{ Kg patient}}{72 \text{ x creat}}$$

8. Know that in **Metabolic Alkalosis**,

   ✪ a <u>Urine Chloride<10</u> **points** to <u>surreptious vomiting</u> **(loss of HCl yields a met alk)**

   ✪ a <u>Urine Chloride>10</u> **points** to <u>Bartter's syndrome</u> and <u>diuretics.</u>

> **Don't confuse:** <u>Laxative abuse,</u> while it will give you a Urine Cl<10, is metabolic *acidosis* 2° to loss of bicarb!

---

9. ✪ Remember, in **Bartter's Syndrome**, because of pathology at the tubules, Na+ is lost, leading to volume loss, which in turn causes ↑renin →↑ aldo→↓K. *The Blood Pressure is low/normal* despite the ↑ renin and ↑ aldo.

10. It might help you to remember one if you know the other since they are practically *opposites* in these regards:

	Type 4 RTA	**Bartter's Syndrome**
Renin	↓	↑
Aldo	↓	↑
K+	↑	↓
BP	↑	↓/normal
Acid-base	Met. **acidosis** (nonAG)	Met. **Alkalosis** (Chloride resistant)

11. Know the electrolyte picture **NSAIDs** can give→↑K+, ↓Na+.

12. Crusty facial lesion followed by nephritis→***Post-Streptococcal Glomerulonephritis***.

13. Know what medicines can *increase your Uric Acid*, such as thiazides and ethanol.

14. ✪ Recognize a case of *E. Coli 0157H7-induced HUS* (Hemolytic Uremic Syndrome) with Anemia; Thrombocytopenia; Renal failure following, e.g., ingested of tainted beef (ATR, which is the middle part of "F**AT R**N" (**F**ever-**A**nemia-**T**hrombocytopenia-**R**enal Failure-**N**eurologic signs), used to help remember the clinical signs of TTP (Thrombotic Thrombocytopenic Purpura)

15. *Acyclovir*→renal intratubular obstruction with crystals.

16. 2 Q's on *Multiple Myeloma*;

   - Know that a *UPEP* (urine protein electropheresis) will do just that and will show any light chains and/or monoclonal IgM spikes.
   - Know that a *dipstick* does not detect light chains, so e.g. you might see only 1+ protein on the dipstick but 23grams of protein on a 24 hour collection!
   - Know that a *low Anion Gap* is consistent with the diagnosis.

17. Remember, in *symptomatic hypovolemic hypoNa+*→the first step is NS (normal saline) even before hypertonic saline, and that the danger of restoring the Na+ too fast is CPM (Central Pontine Myelinolysis).

18. Know the mechanism of **NSAID-induced renal toxicity**:

   a) Renal *prostaglandin inhibition*→↓renal blood flow→prerenal azotemia. This is a *vascular* phenomenon and is the main mechanism of injury for the exam.
   b) ↓Renin→↓aldo→↑K+; =Type 4 RTA

19. Autosomal Dominant Polycystic Kidney Disease (**ADPKD**) is often associated with:

   a) *Cerebral aneurysms* (MRI/MRA not necessary for all ADPKD unless + FH of aneurysm)
   b) *MVP*
   c) Hepatic cysts
   d) Elevated Hct

20. Struvite stones ↔ staghorn calculi ↔ urease-splitting bacteria (e.g. proteus; u.urealyticum).

21. Of all the types of renal stones, Calcium Oxalate stones are the most common, and can result from any of the following aberrations in the urine: ↑Ca (remember to r/o hyperpara); ↑Oxalate, ↑U.A.; or ↓ citrate (usually a protective factor)

22. Uric Acid stones are radiolucent.

23. Remember, a workup for causes of nephrolithiasis or renal stones is indicated for:

   a) Recurrent stones (≥2 stones)
   b) Significant + FH of stones
   c) Young (<25) or older (>60) patients

24. **Commonly Seen Examples of Mixed acid-base disturbances:**

   Combined Acidoses (Resp—1st example + Metabolic-2nd example)
   a) Resp failure + Circulatory failure (lactic acidosis)
   b) Sedatives + ASA
   c) COPD + Renal failure (or sepsis)

   Combined Alkalosis (Resp--1st + Metabolic—2nd)
   - [(Pregnancy or cirrhosis)—hyperventilation] + (diuretics or vomiting)

   Resp Acidosis—1st + Metabolic Alkalosis—2nd
   - COPD + (diuretics or steroids)

   Metabolic Acidosis + Resp Alkalosis
   a) ASA (Resp Alk first then Met Acidosis)
   b) Sepsis (lactic acidosis with secondary resp alk)
   c) Cirrhosis

   Metabolic Acidosis—1st + Metabolic Alkalosis—2nd
   - (Diabetic or alcoholic ketoacidosis) + vomiting

   "Triple Disorder" (combination of the previous 2 categories)
   - (Diabetic or alcoholic ketoacidosis) + (sepsis or cirrhosis)

25. Muddy brown casts → ATN (Acute tubular necrosis)

26. Overview of **Management of Renal Stones by Size**:

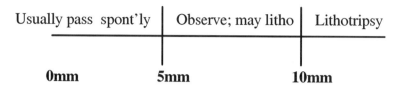

Usually pass spont'ly	Observe; may litho	Lithotripsy
0mm	5mm	10mm

27. **Interstitial nephritis** 2° to drug hypersensitivity→check Hansel's stain for **_urine eosinophils_**.

28. **SLE** may yield any of the following histologies:
    a) normal; b) mesangial; c) focal proliferative; d) diffuse proliferative; and e) membranous.

29. SLE flair up during pregnancy→25% fetal mortality.

30. The #1 cause of **Glomerulonephritis** (GN)and the #1 cause of idiopathic microscopic hematuria is IgA Nephropathy (Berger's Disease)

31. In differentiating **GN following URI**, remember the timing is important:
    a) Poststreptococcal GN occurs 7-21 days later.
    b) IgA Nephropathy occurs within 3 days.

32. *Rhabdomyolysis*: labs: ↑CPK,↑K+, ↑U.A., ↑Phos→↓Ca, and ↑creat may be seen if myoglobinuria develops; if urine dipstick + for heme (Hgb or Mgb) and yet few or no RBCs→suspect myoglobinuric renal failure.

33. *Phosphate levels* <1 mg/dl are truly critical, since life-threatening muscle weakness (cardiac and diaphragmatic) may lead to CHF/ respiratory failure. Hemolysis/rhabdo/ARF may also develop.

34. If you see **RBC casts** → Think *glomerular* nephritis
    "   "   "   **WBC/ WBC casts**→ Think *interstitial* nephritis

35. The **FENa+** (fractional excretion of Na+) is the most helpful urinary index to differentiate prerenal from intrinsic renal failure (<1% vs. >1-3%):

$$\text{FENa} = \frac{\text{clearance of Na+}}{\text{clearance of Creat}} = \frac{\text{Urine}_{Na}/\text{Plasma}_{Na}}{\text{Urine}_{Cr}/\text{Plasma}_{Cr}} = \frac{\text{Urine}_{Na}}{\text{Plasma}_{Na}} \times \frac{\text{Plasma}_{Cr}}{\text{Urine}_{Cr}}$$

36. Both aminoglycoside- and radiocontrast-induced ARF occur 5-7 days after introduction.

37. These are the risk factors for developing **NSAID-induced ARF**:
    a) Preexisting renal insufficiency
    b) Diuretics/volume depletion/hypotension
    c) States of relative intravascular volume depletion (cirrhosis; nephrosis; CHF)
    d) Advanced age

38. Risk factors for **radiocontrast-induced ARF**:

    a) All the above factors for NSAID-induced ARF;
    b) DM with azotemia
    c) Large contrast load or multiple exposures
    d) MM (multiple myeloma) with dehydration

39. Symptoms of ↓K+:

    a) Weakness
    b) Ileus
    c) Polyuria

40. In general, ↑ serum Na+ is 2° to dehydration, and
    ↓ serum Na+ is 2° to fluid overload

41. Therefore, the treatment of *Hyponatremia* 98% of the time is *fluid restriction* (isovolemic—also called euvolemic—and hypervolemic branches of the hyponatremia algorithm). The other 2% is the hypovolemic branch and the treatment of that is either isotonic saline (.95NS) if patient is asymptomatic or hypertonic saline (3% NS) if symptomatic.

42. Laboratory Expressions of Albumin Excretion:

ABNORMAL ALBUMIN EXCRETION RATES BY STYLE OF COLLECTION			
	24-h collection (mg/24h)	Timed collection (ug/min)	Spot collection (ug/mg creatinine)
Normal	<30	<20	<30
Microalbuminuria	30-300	20-200	30-200
Clinical albuminuria	>300	>200	>300

✪ 43. You must know *all* of the following key associations for the following glomerulopathies:

GN		Important Associations
MPGN	→	HepB, SLE, Sickle Cell, ↓C′
Minimal Change Disease	→	Hodgkins Dz, NSAIDs, 80% respond to steroids
Focal Segmental Sclerosis	→	HIV; heroine
Membranous	→	Hep C; Solid organ neoplasms(esp lung, colon). Membranous yields renal vein thrombosis in 25-50% of cases. It is also the #1 cause of idiopathic nephrosis in adults

44. **Know these important causes of ↑K+: "RHABDO":**

    R habdomyolysis

    H emolysis

    A ddison's Disease

    B ad kidneys (ARF, CRF)

    D rugs (ACE I, K+ sparing diuretics)

    O (hyporenin hypoaldo)

45. **Know the DDx for ↓ Mg: "ABCDEFGH":**

    A TN, ↑ Aldo

    B artter Syndrome

    C yclosporin, Cisplatinum

    D iuretics

    E thanol

    F at losses (malabsorption syndromes)

    G astric losses (NG suction, vomiting)

    H ypoparathyroidism

IMPORTANT FIGURES TO LEARN:

ACUTE RENAL FAILURE: *The Big Picture*

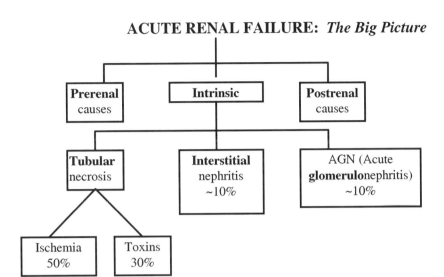

Noteworthy Sediment Analysis in Acute Renal Failure

Prenatal azotemia → Hyaline casts possible
Tubular Injury → Pigmented granular casts
Interstitial nephritis → White cells/white cell casts; eos/eos casts
Glomerulonephritis → Red cells/red cell casts.

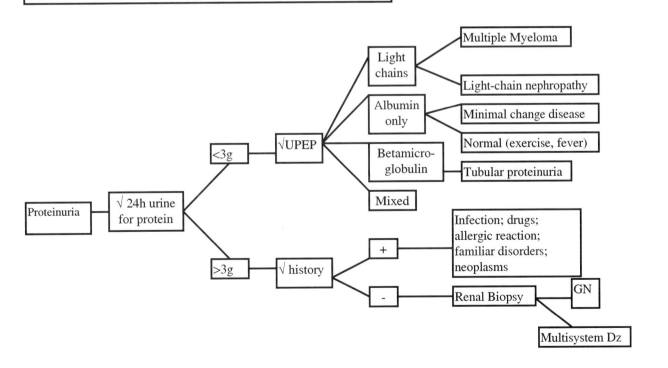

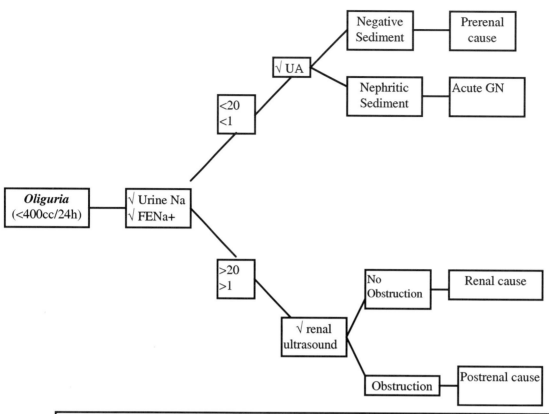

Disorder		Key Implicated Agents to remember
ARF		
Prerenal azotemia	→	NSAIDs; ACEI; radiocontrast
ATN	→	Aminoglycosides; Amphotericin
Intratubular obstruction	→	Acyclovir; Methotrexate
Rhabdomyolysis	→	Lovastatin; Gemfibrozil; heroin
Glomerulonephropathy		
Membranous GN	→	Gold; PCM (Penicillamine)
Focal segmental glomerular sclerosis	→	Heroin
Obstructive Uropathy		
Urolithiasis	→	Allopurinol; Triamterene
Retroperitoneal fibrosis	→	Methylsergide
Vascular or Microvascular Disease		
HUS	→	Mitomycin; Cyclosporin
Tubulointerstitial nephritis		
AIN (Acute Interstitial Nephritis)	→	B-lactam Abx; NSAIDs; sulfonamides; diuretics; rifampin; cimetidine.
Chronic Renal Failure	→	ASA; Acetaminophen
Fluids & Electrolyte disorders		
RTA	→	Amphotericin; outdated TCN
Nephrogenic D.I.	→	Lithium
HyperK+	→	ACE I; NSAIDs; Cyclosporine
HypoNa+	→	NSAIDs; thiazides
HypoMg+	→	Amphotericin; Cisplatin; Aminoglycosides
Hypocalcemia	→	Cisplatin
HypoK+	→	Thiazides; Aminoglycosides

II. CLINICAL PHARMACOLOGY & TOXICOLOGY

Commonly Asked Material:

1. Know that *isopropyl* alcohol (rubbing alcohol) causes ketones, and an osmolar gap but NOT an anion gap.

2. *Anion Gap*= [Na-(HCO3 + Cl)=8-12]

    ✪ *Causes of High Anion Gap* (>12) : **K-U-S-S-M-A-U-L** (Ketoacidosis; Uremia; Starvation; Salicylates; Methanol; Alkali loss; Unusual chemicals; Lactate) ; may use in combination with **C--M-U-D P-I-L-E-S** (Cyanide; Methanol; Uremia; DKA; Paraldehyde/Propylene glycol; INH/Iron; Lactate; Ethylene Glycol; Strychnine/Salicylates/Starvation.)

3. *Osmolar Gap*= 2[Na+] + [Glucose/18] + [BUN/2.8] . Greater than 10 is abnormal.

    -   Osmolar Gap= the measured osmolarity (lab) - your calculated osmolarity

    ✪ Main causes are alcohols (generally end in -**OLS**) ⇒ methan**OL**; ethan**OL**; ethylene glyc**OL**; isopropyl alcoh**OL**; mannit**OL**; and acetone.

    ✪ Know that *ethylene glycol* (antifreeze) gives calcium oxalate crystals.

4. Management of *theophylline toxicity*→ Charcoal lavage and hemodialysis are excellent.
    -   Presentation of theo toxicity→*Cardiac/GI/Neuro* symptoms.

SPECIFIC OVERDOSE SYNDROMES with presentations/mnemonics/management:

ANTICHOLINERGIC SYNDROME (Atropine; TCA's; Antipsychotics; Anthistamines; some Parkinson's meds)

   Presentation—Dry skin and mucous membranes; hyperthermia; flushing;tachycardia; HTN; mydriasis; ↓ salivation and sweating; ileus; urinary retention; anxiety/confusion; seizures.

   ✪ *Mnemonic:* " **Dry as a bone; red as a beet; blind as a bat; mad as a hatter; hot as hades**".

CHOLINERGIC SYNDROME (Organophosphate poisoning)

   Presentation—Essentially the opposite of anticholinergic syndrome, with ↑sweating /salivation/ lacrimation; vomiting; diarrhea; miosis; bradycardia; wheezing; muscle cramps; fasciculations; altered mental status.

   ✪ *Mnemonic*--"**S-L-U-D-G-E**": **S**alivation/sweating; **L**acrimation; **U**rination; **D**efecation; **GI** upset; **E**mesis.

OPIATE OVERDOSE (e.g. morphine, codeine, heroine, methadone)

Presentation—Miosis; *respiratory depression*; drowsiness; N/V; Pulmonary edema; seizures.
   ✪ ***Classic Triad***---↓Mental status; ↓ Respiratory; ↓ pupil size (miosis).

Remember, heroine and methadone may cause ***pulmonary edema***.

BARBITURATES (e.g. phenobarbitol)

Presentation—**all are** ↓: CNS/Resp system/Pulse/BP/Temp/Reflexes

STIMULANTS (amphetamines; cocaine)

Presentation—↑ BP and Pulse and Pupils (mydriasis); CNS agitation/excitation/seizure/
   hallucinations; arrythmias;

SUBSTANCE WITHDRAWAL:

Presentation is as per Stimulants presentation above (minus arrythmias) + N/V/abdominal pain

QUICK PEARLS:

   ✪ Remember, *Naloxone (Narcan)* is used diagnostically in unclear cases to check for opiate
   overdose, and is also used therapeutically (e.g. IV Naloxone drip, since the half-life is extremely
   short relative to the half-life of the opiates).

   • Re: *Anion Gap and Osmolar Gap* are important in toxicology, since having the results of both can
   narrow the cause significantly. Note, for example:

      ✪ *Isopropyl alcohol* (rubbing alcohol) causes an **OG and ketosis, but no AG**.
      ✪ *Methanol and ethylene glycol*, on the other hand, **cause both gaps**.

GASTRIC LAVAGE

   • Before gastric lavage, ***cuffed endotracheal tube*** should be placed if patient has altered mental
   status, depressed gag reflex, or seizures, to prevent aspiration.
   • Activated charcoal treatment of choice for most poisonings (1g/kg)
      • e.g. in *salicylate overdose*, besides activated charcoal…
         1. Fluids important to correct losses and promote diuresis;
         2. Monitor K+ levels;
         3. Alkalinization to increase urinary excretion.
   • Charcoal is generally ineffective in absorbing ***small ionic compounds***, like Lithium, Mg,
   Arsenic, Alcohols (***Hemodialysis*** better for these compounds)
   • Charcoal should not be given for caustic ingestion.

HEMOPERFUSION

- Appropriate for overdoses of phenobarbital; other barbiturates; also theophylline.

✪ *DRUG/TOXIN* → ✪ *ANTIDOTE*

Acetaminophen — N-acetylcysteine (should be given w/in 24h of ingestion: loading dose then q4h x 17 *more* doses)

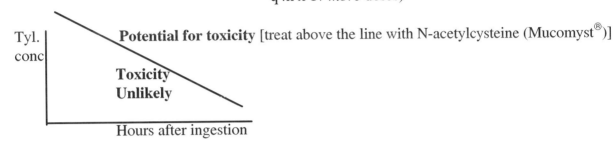

Tyl. conc — **Potential for toxicity** [treat above the line with N-acetylcysteine (Mucomyst®)]

Toxicity Unlikely

Hours after ingestion

Drug/Toxin	Antidote
Anticholinergics	Physostigmine
Benzodiazepines	Flumazenil
Beta-blockers	Glucagon
Carbon monoxide	Oxygen
Cyanide	Amyl nitrite, Na+Nitrite, Na+Thiosulfate
Ethylene Glycol	Ethanol
Iron	Deferoxamine
INH	Pyridoxine
Methanol	Ethanol
Narcotics	Naloxone
Nitrites	Methylene Blue
Organophospates	Atropine, Pralidoxime
TCA's	Na+Bicarbonate

SALICYLATES

- Remember→*charcoal, fluid diuresis, alkalinize the urine*
- Think of OD when you have Resp alkalosis and a High Anion Gap
- Progression is from: *Resp Alkalosis→Resp Alkalosis + Metabolic Acidosis→Metabolic Acidosis*

DIGOXIN

- Atropine often effective for bradycardias
- Lidocaine or Dilantin preferred for Ventricular irritability
- Digoxin-specific Fab fragments (Digibind®) *reserved for severe intoxication*—it binds the Digoxin making it incapable of binding at its receptor, the Na+/K+-ATPase.

TRICYCLIC ANTIDEPRESSANT OVERDOSE:

TCA's: 4 Main Actions→	*Causing:*
1. Quinidine-like effect	↑ PR, QRS, and QT; arrythmias; ↓ BP
2. Anticholinergic	See "Anticholinergic Syndrome" presentation above
3. Block NE reuptake	↓Myocardial contractility; ↓BP and P
4. Antihistamine	--

TRICYCLIC ANTIDEPRESSANT OVERDOSE

- One of the most serious types of OD
- 25% of all deaths due to poisoning
- Deterioration is rapid
- Seizures common
- Activated charcoal
- Do not induce vomiting
- Lidocaine and Dilantin may be used for the ventricular arrythmias
- For ↓BP, avoid Isuprel/Dobutamine/low-dose Dopamine

15.   <u>BLOOD GAS ANALYSIS</u>

IN GENERAL...

See pCO_2 $\longrightarrow$ <u>*Think* Respiratory</u>
(Lungs)

See HCO_3^- $\longrightarrow$ <u>*Think* Metabolic</u>
(Kidneys)

COMPENSATION AXES:

<u>1° Respiratory</u>		<u>2° Metabolic</u>
Acidosis	$\longleftrightarrow$	Alkalosis
Alkalosis	$\longleftrightarrow$	Acidosis

<u>1° Metabolic</u>		<u>2° Respiratory</u>
Acidosis	$\longleftrightarrow$	Alkalosis
Alkalosis	$\longleftrightarrow$	Acidosis

1° **Respiratory Process** (pCO$_2$)

✪ Use Winter's formulas to figure the HCO$_3^-$. Here's our easy quick-chart way:

	HCO$_3^-$		HCO$_3^-$	
ACUTE	↓	60	↓	**CHRONIC**
Resp	+1		+3	Resp
Process		50		Process
	+1		+3	
Normals →	(24)	**40**	(24)	
	-2		-5	
		30		
	-2		-5	
		20		
		↑		
		pCO$_2$		

✪ NOTE that the "+1, +3, -2, and -5" are the amounts that should be added or subtracted from 24 to calculate the true HCO3$^-$, using Winter's formulas, given any pCO$_2$.

✪ If HCO$_3^-$ is more or less than the expected compensation, then there's *another* primary process going on.

WORK THROUGH THESE EXAMPLES :

- If a patient is in <u>ACUTE</u> respiratory distress (see the <u>LEFT SIDE</u> of this Winter's formulas quick-chart), and her pCO2 is 20, you see that the bicarb should be 24-2-2more, which=20! If her bicarb is any more or less, there is *another primary* process going on. If her bicarb is 20, then her bicarb is appropriately compensated and the process is straightforward.

- If a patient is in <u>ACUTE</u> respiratory distress and he becomes lethargic, and his pCO2 is 60, you see that the bicarb should be 24 +1 +1 more, which=26, again if appropriately compensated and assuming no additional contributing process.

- If a patient is in <u>CHRONIC</u> respiratory distress (see the <u>RIGHT SIDE</u> of the Winter's formulas quick-chart), and his pCO2 is 30, you see that the bicarb should be 24 -5, or 19.

- If a patient is in <u>CHRONIC</u> respiratory distress, and his pCO2 is 50, you see that the bicarb should be 24 +3, or 27.

1° Metabolic Process (HCO₃⁻)

If PaO2 ↑s with ↑FIO2, →there's NO SHUNT.

Key examples includes...

1. Asthma
2. Interstitial lung disease
3. Pulmonary Embolus

✪ If PaO2 *does not correct* with↑FIO2→ there *IS* A SHUNT

Intrapulmonary
(more common)

Intracardiac
(less common)

Examples include...

1. Atelectasis
2. ETT down right main bronchus
3. Perfused but unventilated alveoli; alveoli filled with...
   a. Aspiration
   b. Edema
   c. Pus
   d. Blood

Examples include...

1. VSD
2. ASD

Important Tips and Rules of Thumb on ABGs:

- ✪ Whenever see ↓pO2 *plus* ↓pCO2, always calculate the <u>A-a gradient</u>.

- ✪ Whenever see a metabolic acidosis, always calculate the <u>Anion Gap.</u>

- ✪ Whenever see a metabolic alkalosis, know that the next step is to ask for a …
<u>Urine chloride.</u>

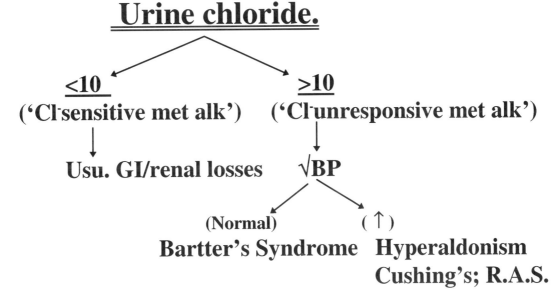

- ✪ Remember, in using the <u>Winter's</u> formulas quick-chart in cases of <u>COPD</u>, remember to refer to the right side of the chart for figuring compensated HCO_3^-.

REMEMBER

Calculating the "Delta-Delta" in Acid-Base Disorders:

✪ *WHAT IS THE DELTA-DELTA ANYWAYS ?!*

- Remember, **delta** also **means "change". The "delta-delta" refers to the change in Anion Gap divided by the change in** HCO_3^- **, or**

$$\boxed{\frac{\Delta\, AG}{\Delta\, HCO_3^-}}$$

- **It should be calculated whenever you have an ↑AG metabolic acidosis. Here's why**...

- Basically, it's done in order to figure out if there's a second underlying disorder, i.e. a **mixed disorder**. In general, for every ↑ in the AG, there is an equal ↓ in the HCO_3^- , so...

- **If the delta-delta<1**, that means there's A "CONCEALED" (or additional hidden) *NON-ANION GAP METABOLIC ACIDOSIS*. Why? Because < 1 implies that the change in the bicarb was greater than the change in the AG. That means the ↓ in bicarb was more than expected for the anion gap alone.

- **If the delta-delta is > 1**, that means there's a CONCEALED *METABOLIC ALKALOSIS*. The logic is the same.

✪ **FOR EXAMPLE, given the upper limit of a normal AG is 12, if the** patient's AG = 20, the Δ AG therefore =8, so we'd expect a Δ HCO_3^- to be the same, or (24-X) = 8, so "X", or the measured HCO_3^- we would *expect to be* 16. If it's > 16, the delta-delta will be >1, and there must be a concealed metabolic alkalosis. Perhaps the patient has been vomiting too (losing acid) ? If the measured HCO_3^- <16, the delta-delta <1, so there must be an additional or concealed non-anion gap metabolic acidosis.

REMEMBER TOO:

- ✪ Acidemia ———————→ Hyperkalemia
- ✪ Alkalemia ———————→ Hypokalemia

- ✪ The #1 cause of hypoxemia is *hypoventilation*

- ✪ ↑A-a gradient means <u>abnormal lung!</u>

- If you see a ↓PaO2, ↓sat (lab), normal pulse ox, and patient is non-cyanotic, think→<u>Leukocyte larceny</u> (occurs in the lab)

- If you see ↓sat, cyanotic patient, and normal PaO2, think→<u>Methemoglobinemia</u> (congenital right-shifted hemoglobin)

- If you see sat % unusually/inappropriately high for the level of PaO2, think→<u>Cyanide or carboxyHg</u> (common in firefighters)

Blood Gases APPENDIX
Key Formulas; DDx; & Compensation

Anion Gap: $[Na^+ - (HCO_3+Cl)] = 8-12$ (normal range)

- Causes of High Anion Gap (>12) : **K-U-S-S-M-A-U-L** (Ketoacidosis; Uremia; Starvation; Salicylates; Methanol; Alkali loss; Unusual chemicals; Lactate) ; **OR**...

- **C--M-U-D P-I-L-E-S** (Cyanide; Methanol; Uremia; DKA; Paraldehyde/Propylene glycol; INH/Iron Lactate; Ethylene Glycol; Strychnine/Salicylates/Starvation.)

Osmolar Gap $= 2[Na+] + [Glucose/18] + [BUN/2.8]$. Greater than 10 is abnormal.

- Osmolar Gap= the measured osmolarity (lab) - your calculated osmolarity

- Main causes end in -**OLS**: Methan**OL**; Ethan**OL**; Ethylene Glyc**OL**; Isopropyl Alcoh**OL**; Mannit**OL**; and acetone.

✪ A-a Gradient $= pAO_2-paO_2 = [150 - \dfrac{pCO2}{0.8}] - paO2$

DDx of ↑A-a (Alveolar-arterial) Gradient→Remember, "VSD"
1. **V**/Q mismatching, e.g.
   a. PE
   b. Airway obstruction
2. **S**hunt
   a. Intracardiac (e.g. VSD!)
   b. Intrapulmonary (ARDS, CHF)
3. **D**iffusion defect, e.g.
   a. IPF (idiopathic pulmonary fibrosis)
   b. Emphysema

✪ Calculating Compensation

- **Metabolic acidosis→ $pCO_2=1.5 (HCO_3^-) + 8 \pm 2$**

- **Metabolic alkalosis→pCO2 last 2 digits ≈ last 2 digits of the pH (that's an easy calculation!)**

- **Respiratory acidosis/alkalosis→HCO3⁻ as per our Winter's formulas quick-chart**

16. <u>STATISTICS</u>

IT'S ALL ABOUT...
- Knowing how to set up your "2 by 2" table
- Knowing the terms and equations
- Knowing the pattern of solving these questions
- Let's walk through it...

ALWAYS SET UP YOUR 2X2 TABLE THIS WAY:

	DISEASE PRESENT	**DISEASE ABSENT**
DIAGNOSTIC TEST +	True + "a"	False + "b"
DIAGNOSTIC TEST -	False - "c"	True - "d"

IMPORTANT NOTES:

- ✪ *Don't put the headings on the wrong axis !!*
- ✪ **The most important players are "a" and "d"**—remember their position!
- ✪ **Sensitivity** goes <u>down the 1st column</u>!
- ✪ **Specificity** goes <u>down the 2nd column</u>!
- ✪ **Positive Predictive Value (PPV)** goes <u>across the 1st row</u>!
- ✪ **Negative Predictive Value (NPV)** goes <u>across the 2nd row</u>!

SO, SETTING IT UP AGAIN spatially MUCH SIMPLER THIS TIME IT GOES LIKE THIS:
{placement of capitals to illustrate relative importance}

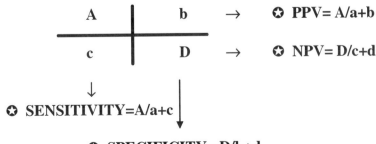

| A | b | → | ✪ PPV= A/a+b |
| c | D | → | ✪ NPV= D/c+d |

✪ **SENSITIVITY=A/a+c**

✪ **SPECIFICITY= D/b+d**

✪ And **PREVALENCE= a+c/a+b+c+d**

SO! Let's Do An <u>EXAMPLE</u> In A Manner Commonly Presented...

- You're given a new diagnostic test that gives abnormal results 80% of patients who have the disease but gives normal results in 95% of patients who are truly disease-free. We also tell you that the prevalence of the disease in the population being tested is 10%. Now let's say you're asked what % of patients who test + actually have the disease (asking Positive Predictive Value).

WE NOW HAVE EVERYTHING WE NEED:

1. Sensitivity = 80%
2. Specificity = 95%
3. Prevalence = 10%

...which is everything we need to set up our 2x2 table and fill in the blanks.

<u>**IMPORTANT**</u>: *The key to solving these problems is <u>the order in which you proceed</u>.*
(I've charted the itinerary for you)

FIRST: <u>Start with the prevalence</u> and arbitrarily assume a population of 100;
Well, that means a+b+c+d=100; so 10% of that population the prevalence.

SECOND: That means <u>a+c</u> =10, since those are the ones who actually have the disease.

THIRD: So, we start picking them off one at a time. If a+c=10, and the <u>sensitivity</u> is 80%, that means <u>"a" must = 8</u>; and therefore <u>"c" must =2</u>. Remember, we're setting this all up so we can calculate the PPV in *percent (!) so don't worry.*

FOURTH: <u>100 minus 10 (which was a+c, remember) gives us 90, which must = b+d</u>. Now we punch in the <u>specificity</u>, which is 95%, so d/b+d, or d/90=95%. That means <u>"d"= 85.5</u> (don't worry that's 855 if you arbitrarily chose a population of 1000), so <u>"b" must =</u> 90-85.5=4.5

FINALLY: <u>So, we now have all the values for "a","b","c", and "d", and we can calculate either PPV or NPV, whatever is asked</u>. Our example asked for PPV, so that's a/a+b, or 8/8+4.5, (or 80/80+45, if you chose to use 1000), so...

<u>PPV=64%</u>, and that's the answer you look for!

INDEX

D

E

F

I

J

K

Q

REFERENCES

1. Harrison's Principles of Internal Medicine 15th edition, McGraw Hill Inc., New York, © 2001 by McGraw Hill Inc.
2. Pretest Self Assessment and Review-Harrison's Principles of Internal Medicine, 14th ed, Richard M. Stone et al, McGraw Hill Inc., New York, © 1998.
3. Cecil Essentials of Medicine, 5th edition, Andreoli, T. et al, W. B. Saunders Company, Philadelphia, PA © 2000.
4. Frontrunners Internal Medicine Board Review Course, 1996-2001.
5. Frontrunners Q&A Review for the I.M. Boards: 1234 Questions & Answers to Prepare You, Mittman, B., Frontrunners Board Review, Inc., Bayside, NY, © 2001
6. Mayo Internal Medicine Board Review, Udaya B.S. Prakash (ed), Mayo Foundation for Medical Education and Research, Rochester, MN, © 2000-2001.
7. ACP Board Review Course, 1996-2001.
8. Emory University Comprehensive Board Review in Internal Medicine
9. Medical Knowledge Self Assessment Program VII, VIII, IX, X, XI, and XII, American College of Physicians, Philadelphia, PA.
10. Heart Disease- A Textbook of Cardiovascular Medicine, edited by Eugene Braunwald, MD, 5th ed, W.B. Saunders Company, © 2000
11. The Sanford Guide to Antimicrobial Therapy 2000, David N. Gilbert, MD, et al, 30th ed., © 2001.

Quick Order Form

We ALSO provide these additional I.M. board review resources:

❑ *Frontrunners Q&A Review for the I.M. Boards* : **1234 Questions & Answers...**

❑ Frontrunners **Weekend Marathon Review** (for the ABIM Exam): certification & recertification (call 888-440-2246 for dates/details)

❑ Intensive 4 month Internal Medicine Board Review Course (call for dates/details)

ORDER OPTIONS: **(check off any of the above; if requesting info only, use this form and just say so ☺)**

Fax orders: **516-977-3294**. Fax this form.

Tel. Orders: Call **888-440-ABIM (2246)**. Credit card may be securely left here. V/MC/AmX only.

E-mail orders: Order details may also be emailed to us at **abimexam@aol.com**

Order *by mail*: Frontrunners Board Review, Inc.
Attention: Orders Department
39 Lyon St.
Valley Stream, NY 11580

CUSTOMER: _____

Address: _____

City State Zip: _____

Fax # (to be used for faxback confirmation only!): _____

PAYMENT: ❑ Check ❑ Visa ❑ MC ❑ AmX

Card number: _____

Name on card: _____Exp. Date _____

Quick Order Form

We ALSO provide these additional I.M. board review resources:

☐ *Frontrunners Q&A Review for the I.M. Boards* : **1234 Questions & Answers...**

☐ Frontrunners **Weekend Marathon Review** (for the ABIM Exam): certification & recertification (call 888-440-2246 for dates/details)

☐ Intensive 4 month Internal Medicine Board Review Course (call for dates/details)

ORDER OPTIONS: **(check off any of the above; if requesting info only, use this form and just say so ☺)**

Fax orders: **516-977-3294**. Fax this form.

Tel. Orders: Call **888-440-ABIM (2246)**. Credit card may be securely left here. V/MC/AmX only.

E-mail orders: Order details may also be emailed to us at **abimexam@aol.com**

Order *by mail*: Frontrunners Board Review, Inc.
Attention: Orders Department
39 Lyon St.
Valley Stream, NY 11580

CUSTOMER: _____

Address: _____

City State Zip: _____

Fax # (to be used for faxback confirmation only!): _____

PAYMENT: ☐ Check   ☐ Visa   ☐ MC   ☐ AmX

Card number: _____

Name on card: _____ Exp. Date _____